The Smart GI Diet Plan

Kim G. Bryan

Kim G Bryan

ACKNOWLEDGEMENTS

This book would not have been possible without the help and support of many people.

My family, especially my wonderful sister, Dr. Christine Bryan.

My clients, who include English teachers, nurses, chefs and many more!

Zoë Farmer, for all her excellent graphics.

And finally,
Shona Ross, my friend and colleague for all her ideas, she is a constant source of inspiration.

The Smart GI Diet Plan

CONTENTS

Preface

The Smart GI Diet Plan

PREFACE

Ten years have passed since I wrote the first edition of this book and within that time the subject of sugar and its destruction on the human body has become extremely topical.

Numerous studies have been carried out and the conclusions are always the same "too much sugar is bad". The majority of you will believe this is a new and modern phenomenon but a British Professor back in 1972 predicted the sugar boom and the destruction it would bring.

John Yudkin had actually predicted the problems with sugar in his book 'Pure, White and Deadly'.

The publication was scarily prophetic of what we are now experiencing and actually led to the end of his career. By the end of the 70's he was totally discredited and as a result the low fat diet crazes boomed.

An excessive amount of fat is probably not the healthiest option but fat is not necessarily the enemy here.

Sugar, which is hidden in abundance in often the most innocent looking foods is enemy no.1 and as a result it will as Professor Yudkin predicted, destroy us!

The Smart GI Diet Plan

INTRODUCTION

The amount of people who are overweight and clinically obese is increasing. It is a fact that one in four people are now classed as obese in the United Kingdom. Unfortunately, these figures now include children. People get caught up in a vicious circle, starting the latest 'fad diets' in a hope to lose all their excess weight in the fastest possible time. Certain 'fad diets' promise miraculous results. These results never happen and people end up very depressed with a zapped self-confidence and feel that they are destined to be fat forever.

Not everybody can become a 'perfect ten'. Body shape and build differs between individuals. Personalizing your own individual and achievable target is the first step to success. The next step is to commence an eating plan that will be followed for life. A plan that will allow you to enjoy life, gain health and restore a good relationship with food.

The glycaemic index (GI) is a breakthrough in weight control. GI should not be confused with low carbohydrate regimes. Low GI concentrates on the quality of carbohydrate and the concentration of carbohydrate within certain foods, known as glycaemic load.

Unfortunately, there have been some misunderstandings associated with GI with various literatures contradicting each other.

"Carrots make you fat!"

"You can only eat certain foods"

This book explains how to use the whole concept of GI in a simple and user-friendly format.

The SMART GI diet plan has been written with the real person in mind.

Ordinary foods for everyday people.

Dr. Christine Bryan says, "It's not rocket science. It's rocket fuel!"

We look after our cars, regular maintenance, MOT's and using quality fuel for maximum performance. Yet we expect our bodies to function efficiently no matter what!

We may think that we feel o.k.

A change to a lifestyle which includes more exercise and a considered dietary intake and we can feel much healthier.

Learning about the GI values of everyday foods is a good place to start.

WHY ARE YOU OVERWEIGHT?

This question is the first and most important. You can only correct something when you realise why it is wrong.

> - **Over eating?**
> - **Idleness?**
> - **Medical?**
> - **Psychological?**

A person is obese when they are carrying more than 10% of their ideal bodyweight. Ideal body weight varies from person to person and can be determined by having a healthy score (between 20-25) on the Body Mass Index Chart. A person who is 10% over their ideal body weight is overweight.

Check your BMI on the next page.

BMI is an internationally recognised formula.

BMI between 20-25   normal body weight
BMI between 25-30   overweight
BMI between 35-40   obese
BMI over 40   dangerously obese

Normal body weight can fluctuate within a specific range, which allows for different body shapes.

Body Mass Index

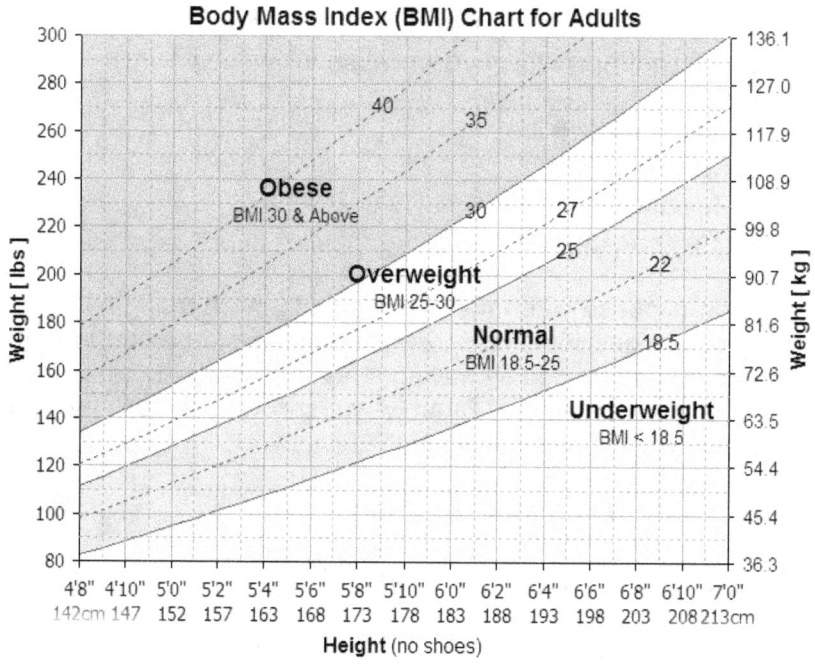

WHY DO YOU WANT TO LOSE WEIGHT?

To be thin? To fit in? To look good in the current fashion? Or maybe, for your health?

Each individual will have a specific reason for losing weight and what may be important to one person will be bottom of the list for others.

Before you embark on a weight reduction programme you must answer the above question very honestly.

Once we set clear goals and understand not only the reason for wanting to lose weight but also the reason why we put the weight on in the first place!

Here are a few examples why people need to start a 'diet'.

> **Getting Married**

This is probably the most important day in any person's life. They need to look fabulous and this means slim! It is quite a sad, but true fact that many brides will do anything to fit into their wonderful wedding gown and then, after the honeymoon, gradually put all their lost weight back on accompanied with a little more! This is apparent with other small occasions e.g. Christmas, holidays or a Summer Ball.

> **Fashion**

Fashion has always dictated how people 'ought' to look. It still does. Fashion clothes seem to be designed to fit a particular body shape, the most suitable models achieve super-model star status and women are 'persuaded' into thinking that this must be the 'perfect body shape'.

➢ Peer pressure

Everybody needs to fit in. The overweight person would feel 'out of place' within a group of slimmer friends, although they never actually admit to this. The dieting culture can become addictive amongst friends. A new 'fad' diet evolves and everybody has to start it. After a few weeks, when the supermodel figure has not been achieved, people give up and eventually the whole group of friends will all give up.

➢ A single comment

A comment like "You've put some weight on" can be the only trigger a person needs. After you have studied yourself in the mirror and eventually come to terms with the fact that the comment was actually true. A comment like this can also have a devastating effect on your self-esteem.

➢ Attracting the opposite sex

The desire to lose weight becomes very strong when we are attempting to attract a mate! Even stronger becomes the desire when we meet somebody and the relationship is new. The thought of our bodies devoid of clothes and exposing all the wobbly bits gives us concern to slim down a little.

➢ Health

This may be the bottom of the list here but it should be top of everybody's list. Health is paramount and being overweight or obese has many problems associated with health and well being.

The Doctor has told you to lose weight because:

- ➢ **You have high cholesterol**
- ➢ **High blood pressure**

> ➢ **Diabetes**
> ➢ **Painful arthritis**
> ➢ **Risk of a heart attack**
> ➢ **Degenerating joints**
> ➢ **All of the above**

Most people want to lose weight for one reason or other reasons and it is likely that they will have several reasons. A number of factors seem to come together at one time, all of which have probably given the individual cause to think about losing their excess weight. One single factor will dominate over the others and that will trigger the need to lose weight.

Once you come to terms with the real reason for losing weight and have this reason set out clearly in your mind that is your first step to success.

DIETRY MISCONSEPTIONS

Many people will have a list of excuses why they are unable to lose weight. These excuses sound so plausible to the individuals but are common dietary misconceptions that are used as a barrier from the truth.

Here is a list of the most common misconceptions.

Do you recognise any of these sayings?

THE FAT GENE RUNS IN OUR FAMILY

The parents of certain overweight people are probably overweight themselves and it would seem that it was all down to genetics. The explanation is more likely to be the eating habits of the person. Bad habits can start when very young, as people tend to trust their parents judgement with regard to food. It is a very sad affair when I observe such people shopping in the supermarket. Their trolleys are full of high fat, processed food, sweets and high sugar fizzy drinks. Any food that would be classed as healthy eating is sadly missing from their trolleys.

IT'S A GLANDULAR PROBLEM

People believe their thyroid gland is not working properly and become quite happy with this excuse. Under-active thyroids are commonplace nowadays but treatable with the correct tests and medication. This misconception is used as an immediate protective barrier for the overweight person. The thyroid blood test could show there was no problem but conditions are hard to erase from peoples minds. To them it is reality.

HOW CAN I BE FAT I EAT VERY LITTLE

People who eat very little are probably eating all the wrong foods throughout the day e.g. chocolate bars, crisps, muffins etc. These foods are convenience foods, high in calories and high in sugar and fat. The total calorie intake totals more than the individuals daily need hence weight gain. These people are unaware of the calorific values of convenience foods and consider these foods as small snacks taking account of the short time it takes to eat them.

I ONLY HAVE TO LOOK AT A CREAM CAKE AND I PUT ON WEIGHT

The sheer fact that these people mention cream cakes denotes that they do actually eat them.

You have to consume food to put on weight!

I'M OK THROUGHOUT THE DAY, I CAN STARVE ALL DAY UNTIL THE EVENING, THEN I HAVE TO EAT OR I FEEL FAINT.

People think that starving is an efficient method for losing weight. If you take nothing in, then you are bound to lose weight. Weight that is lost this way is usually water and muscle mass. The trouble comes when you eat again and this tends to be either the wrong foods, large amounts of food or even worse, both!

After starving, the body goes into metabolic conservation. In layman terms this means that it stores the food rather than using it for energy.

A SMALL CHOCOLATE BAR WON'T HURT. YOU BURN OFF ENERGY QUICKLY.

This depends whether you have one chocolate bar a day or one a week! Some chocolate bars contain as much energy as a complete meal. The trouble is that they are eaten swiftly and then forgotten until you try an item of clothing on that suddenly seems to have shrunk!

MUSCLE IS HEAVIER THAT FAT, SO WHY BOTHER WITH EXERCISE!

Exercise does not turn fat into muscle. Exercise helps to burn off fat and enables the body to build muscle. Muscle may weigh more than fat but it takes up less room. This explains why certain people can drop a dress size without changing weight.

WHY FIGHT NATURE

Nature never intended the human race to be overweight. Everybody has different shapes e.g. wider hips (pelvic bones structure). On the other hand, nature did not intend for us to eat copious amounts of food. Food is merely a fuel for energy and a transport system for nutrition. If nature intended people to be fat then the state of fatness would be associated with better health.

MY METABOLISM IS SLOW

Most people have a normal metabolism. This excuse is used as a protective barrier because it denotes the problem is medical and it is not easy to argue with. Regular healthy eating coupled with moderate exercise will raise metabolic rates but this excuse usually covers the simple fact that they eat too much.

SELF-ESTEEM

Embarking on a new weight loss plan without addressing and analysing our self-esteem is a recipe for failure.

The core of the problem often lies with the fact that self-esteem is unstable.

Imagine self-esteem as the foundations of a house. Is it firm and solid like concrete or is it built on shifting, shaky sands?

Self-esteem is a component part of our self-image.

Self image is broken down into five parts.

- **Self-identity**   **- this is who we think we are**
- **Ideal self**   **- who we would like to be**
- **Social self**   **- whom we are when with others private/public selves**
- **Public**   **- how we show ourselves to the outside world**
- **Private**   **- an inward privacy**

Self-esteem – a personal judgement of our self value

A flagging self-esteem reveals itself as:-

- **Dependency**
- **Constant need for approval**
- **Helplessness**
- **Anxiety**
- **Poor health**
- **Isolation**
- **Depression**

Self-esteem is constantly changing throughout life and life's ups and downs. It can be high one minute and then knocked down the next by external factors e.g. negative comments or losing a job.

You need to determine how your self-esteem rates and how you can change it. Certain experiences in life need to be tackled by a trained counsellor. Example: sexual abuse or abuse from parents.

If the problem lies with negativity and a constant feeling of failure you need to talk to your subconscious mind. Weight reduction and control is not about the food we eat and the exercise we do.

Reducing weight and keeping it off requires personal motivation and specific mental attitudes.

Staying slim is a skill that some people have naturally – but anyone can learn it. It all depends how much you want to be slim opposed to eating unnecessarily. The power of the mind is probably the strongest tool you have in a weight reduction programme.

"A slim mind creates a slim body"

If you constantly flood your mind with negative feeling about yourself you will inevitably fail.

"I am destined to be overweight, it's in my gene"

"I will never be able to stick to it"

"It will work for you but it won't for me"

How about changing this?

"I can do it, I will change my lifestyle and succeed"

"Small changes will make big results"

"I am not going to be overweight anymore"

If you think of yourself as a slimmer person, the subconscious mind will do everything in its power to make it a reality.

Visualise your goals and aspirations. Imagine yourself wearing clothes that you have always wanted to wear. Develop a strong mental picture of yourself because unless you change your body image from fat to slim, you will never make a permanent change in your physical body and you will be overweight forever.

With a clear mental attitude on board you will then need a degree of motivation.

Motivate, Initiate and Succeed!

Remember these three words and remember that they always come in this order.

> ➢ **We cannot start anything without motivation**
> ➢ **Once motivation has set in starting is easy**
> ➢ **Keep on track and success will be yours**

Motivation is probably the missing link for many people. I will start tomorrow or after the Christmas break! The most important thing to remember is motivation come from you. Nobody else can do it for you and the responsibility lies solely upon you.

Family and friends will be supportive but they cannot be held responsible for motivation. Maybe they have promised to buy you an item of clothing if you lose the excess weight.

Motivate and succeed and you can buy your own wardrobe full of clothes.

Motivation comes from you!

"The great dividing line between success and failure can be expressed in five words. 'I did not have time'."

Franklin Field

THE DANGERS OF DIETING!

Over the years there have been so many diets created. These diets become very popular, everybody gets on the bandwagon and yet, the nation is steadily getting bigger!

In fact, obesity figures are now so high and sadly getting higher.

CRASH DIETING

These diets have materialised in many forms. Firstly, starving yourself by skipping meals! To lose weight you must first cut calories. This statement is correct but how people perceive it is quite frightening.

"OK, so all I need to do is cut my calories and I will lose my excess weight."

"I know, I'll severely cut my food intake to about 800 calories a day and I'll lose my weight in a month and then I can eat something good again!"

We all know people who have done this!

Companies sell meal replacement products to make meal times easier. Weight does fall quite dramatically in the early stages but with consequences. Initially, the body loses water, muscle mass and a small proportion of the weight loss will be fat. The body needs energy to survive and it will take energy from whatever source is available. Along with muscle tissue, the body can break down bone and vital organs. Crash diets cannot be maintained for long periods of time, the body is far too intelligent for that to happen.

ANTI-STARVATION TRIGGER

The body is very intelligent. If we work against the natural design, problems will occur. I am sure you have all tried the 'eat like a pigeon diet'? Eat crisp bread and feel very self-righteous for doing so. My stomach is rumbling so I must be losing weight! The trouble with eating like this is the motion of the anti-starvation trigger. This mechanism will be activated if we eat very little and there is nothing we can do to stop it. The body views this eating regime as starvation and when food is available, we inevitably binge. The brain may be saying *"I need to lose weight"* but the body does not respond.

WEIGHT GAIN AFTER A CRASH DIET

The explanation for this is quite simple. If we lower our food intake dramatically, metabolism will automatically lower to compensate. After a while, the anti-starvation trigger takes over and we reward it with large amounts of food. Large food intake with a slower metabolism inevitably ends weight gain.

If we continue to crash diet, binge, crash diet and binge again we will end up heavier than when we initially started. You need to step off the yo-yo dieting treadmill for good.

CALORIE COUNTING

[Reference 1]
A little kinder than crash dieting is a low-calorie diet. Again, people try and speed up the process by conserving and exercising more. Patrick Holford (1999) believes that the maths behind the theory is patently wrong.

Patrick cleverly sums up how counterproductive calorie counting is in the following example.

"A banana is approximately 100 calories, so if you eat one banana less every day for a year you'd lose 36,500 calories. One pound of body fat is equivalent to around 4000 calories.

That means you'd lose 10lb in the first year, 50lb in the fifth year! All by eating one less banana a day. The calories equation for exercise is equally ridiculous. Cycle vigorously for 15 minutes each day and you will lose 10lb in the first year. Quite possible. But 100lb after 10 years? No chance. However, according to calorie theory, a banana everyday undoes all that hard work anyway!"

The calorie theory fails to add up because of a missing link in the equation: metabolism.

LOW FAT DIETS

Walk into any supermarket and you will be bombarded with numerous low fat products. Low fat diets became very popular a few years ago and manufacturers soon set about a task to produce hundreds of low fat products. Products, can be labelled, 'low fat', 'fat free' or '99% fat free' etc. Unfortunately the fat is replaced by other ingredients, mainly sugar as it is cheap and a good product filler. Look at a low fat product and you will convince yourself that eating two will be acceptable.

Certain fats are needed for the body to function efficiently. Fat is needed for healthy skin, lungs and general well being. We should focus on cutting down on saturated fat in our diet but also including various good fats.

Fats are not created equal. There's good, bad and downright ugly! Fat will be explained in full later.

HIGH PROTEIN DIETS

These diets advocate cutting carbohydrates from your diet. The popular Atkins diet advises that in stage one, 20g of carbohydrates should be eaten daily. Protein and fat can be eaten quite liberally. Bacon and eggs for breakfast, lovely! Weight drops very quickly and this aspect has made high protein diets very popular.

The body holds fuel, known as glycogen in the liver and muscles. This fuel is needed to convert glycogen into glucose whenever needed. When the body is starved of carbohydrate it uses up the fuel reserves from the liver and muscles. An average of 11lb of glycogen is held in the human body; hence the dramatic weight loss and also the re-appearance of that weight very quickly when carbohydrates are consumed again. Using protein as a fuel causes the body to form toxic substances called ketones. Increased levels of ketones cause ketosis, a toxic state which is harmful to the body. Ketosis has some nasty side effects: bad breath and lack of energy. Another problem is the protein has to be neutralised by the body. Calcium is released from the bones via urine increasing the risk of osteoporosis.

MAGIC SLIMMING PILLS

Every year, a new pill or potion claims to do it all for you. Have you ever sat back and thought if these products really worked, there would be no overweight people left!

Leaflets drop through the door stating amazing fat loss in a short space of time, just by taking a few pills! People will be walking down the street and losing their clothes! I don't think so.

HOW THE BODY VIEWS HUNGER

The total food intake is determined by our appetite mechanisms.

If no food has been eaten for a few hours your stomach will let you know by gnawing contractions known as hunger pangs. Appetite mechanisms also stimulate parts of our brains. The brain sends a signal, which is quite easily translated to:

"You must search for food to eat!"

At this point, the brain also will determine whether we eat enough or over eat. This is known as disinhibition. If you have a low level of disinhibition you find it easy to stop eating opposed to a person with a high level. These people tend to overeat.

Disinhibition can be controlled by many factors:

> **Choice of food**
> **Regularity of meal**
> **Positive attitude**
> **Psychological control**
> **Happy or sad**
> **Family eating patterns**
> **A combination of the above**

BALANCE BLOOD SUGAR
AND BALANCE YOUR LIFE!

If ever there was a balance that was of crucial importance, it is your blood sugar balance.

Most dieters will know the feeling of low blood sugar.

> **Dizzy**
> **Shaky**
> **Light headed**
> **Angry**
> **Irritability**
> **Confused**
> **Forgetful**
> **Aggressive**
> **Tired**

If all those feelings weren't bad enough, the aftermath of low blood sugar is a headache!

Low blood sugar, known as hypoglycaemia is the result of the body's glucose level falling too low. The body tries to compensate for this by releasing the hormone adrenaline from the adrenal glands and glucagon is produced from the pancreas. Glucagon increases blood glucose by encouraging the liver to convert its glycogen stores into glucose, basically for instant energy

Repeated episodes of this result in hypoglycaemic (low blood sugar level) and can create many problems to a persons health.

The opposite of this is hyperglycaemia (high blood sugar) and this can cause the onset of diabetes. When glucose levels are too high the pancreas, to stabilise glucose to a normal level, produces insulin. Certain people are predisposed to diabetes and there are many people who are putting themselves at risk from the disease without even knowing it.

How do you know if your blood sugar is fluctuating?

> ➢ **Do you find it hard to wake up in the morning?**
> ➢ **Do you need a stimulant to help you wake up e.g. coffee?**
> ➢ **Do you crave refined carbohydrates i.e. sugar, bread etc?**
> ➢ **Do you drink alcohol most days?**
> ➢ **Do you have mood swings?**
> ➢ **Do you get irritable when you go without food?**
> ➢ **Do you often get stressed?**
> ➢ **Do you get angry and aggressive outbursts?**
> ➢ **Do you have low energy levels?**
> ➢ **Do you get daily headaches?**

If you have a few of the above symptoms it is quite likely that your blood sugar fluctuates excessively within a normal day.

Main Reasons

> ➢ **You often skip meals and more often than not, breakfast.**
> ➢ **You reach for a quick fix when you are hungry and not a nutritious meal.**
> ➢ **You go for long periods of time without food.**
> ➢ **When your are over hungry you eat large amounts of refined foods.**
> ➢ **Your meals are lacking vital nutrients.**

Carbohydrates have the greatest effect on blood sugar, as they are our main energy food. Simply cutting them out completely is not the answer as they are not all created equal. Some are bad and some are good but it's getting the balance right that matters. This is where the glycaemic index and glycaemic loads play a vital role.

Fact: raised insulin levels encourage fat storage and discourage the body from burning stored fat.

During a normal day the amount by which our blood sugar fluctuates depends on what we eat, when we eat and the exercise we do.

THE GLYCAEMIC INDEX

[Reference 3]
The glycaemic index is a list of foods, which measure impact on blood sugar balance. Foods are measured against glucose, which has a score of 100. Glucose is a fast releasing carbohydrate and raises insulin to the highest level. Other foods are slow releasing and have a lesser impact on blood sugar balance; insulin levels are lower. Certain factors within food, other than carbohydrate, determine whether a food is 'fast' or 'slow' releasing. The presence of protein, fibre and fat in a food lowers the glycaemic index and has a lesser impact on blood sugar. Example: fruit juice has a higher score because the fibrous fruit (peel) has been taken away. Pulses are high in protein and fibre hence they score very low. The fat content of food will lower the GI of a food but this does not mean you can eat liberal amounts.

In the diet plan you will see that the food lists have been simplified to make your new regime as easy as possible.

Foods that have a low glycaemic index will sustain you for longer and keep hunger at bay. Low GI foods help you burn more body fat opposed to muscle mass.

Only foods that contain carbohydrate can be tested for GI. Protein and fats will be explained in full in the diet plan.

GLYCAEMIC LOAD

[Reference 4]
A very important factor about adopting a low GI diet is the concentration of carbohydrate within a food. This is the amount of carbohydrate that is contained within a food and is known as the glycaemic load. Certain low GI foods have a high concentration of carbohydrate and certain high GI foods have a small quantity.

The GI indicates the impact a food will have on blood glucose levels, whereas the GL denote the power of the impact!

Unfortunately, GI has been perceived as a complicated diet for this reason. Various literatures on the subject contradict the healthiness of certain foods.

EXAMPLES

Watermelon scores 72 on the glycaemic index, its carbohydrate content per 100g is approximately 6g. The glycaemic load works out to 4, which in layman terms is low!

Poor innocent watermelon, which is so refreshing on a hot summer's day, labelled as a fattening food! NONSENSE!

Other fruit and vegetables have been labelled the same way e.g. carrots.

Fruit and vegetables are a very important part of a diet and sadly, many people do not include enough in their diet. The recommendation is to eat at LEAST five portions per day. They provide fibre, vitamins and minerals, which are paramount for good health.

On the opposite end to this are low GI foods, which have high carbohydrate contents. These foods need not be omitted from a diet; just concentrate on the portion size, what you eat with them and when you eat them and food can be enjoyed.

Pasta is a good example here. Heralded a princely, healthy food a few years ago. What did people do? Eat loads of it! The carbohydrate content will vary depending on cooking time but portion size and meal choice is the main problem. There is no need to get confused as the diet plan has been simplified for you.

When I began to research the glycaemic index 2003 certain questions popped up in mind so I decided to ask an expert whose knowledge was second to none.

"The experts never intended the glycaemic index to be used in isolation."

They also urge that people do not make the mistake of using the glycaemic load alone.

This equates to a diet too low in carbohydrate and too high in fat.

Don't worry; the SMART GI diet plan has worked out everything for you from best food choices to an average portion size.

High GI foods are generally foods that have been processed

and refined with various ingredients added.

EXAMPLES

White bread	Chocolate bars
Bagels	Pastries
French baguettes	Sausage rolls
Sugary breakfast cereals	Doughnuts
Refined fruit juice	Fizzy drinks
White rice	Potato crisps
Biscuits and wafers	Sweets
Processed quick meals	Cakes

We all like to treat ourselves to one or two of the above list from time to time and that is OK. The trouble is, for many of the population, the above list is their staple diet!

The SMART GI diet plan will show you how making a few changes to your diet can help balance the body's blood sugar, encourage the body to burn stored fat and obtain optimum health.

BACK TO BASICS

Ok, so you've tried all the latest diets; high protein, no protein, low carbohydrate, no carbohydrate after a certain time and then you hear that the best diets are the ones that do not omit any food groups. Confused?

Many people have no idea about nutrition and why we need to eat certain foods or even worse, they do not know which foods fall in which category!

A BRIEF GUIDE TO NUTRITION

Essential nutrients are classified as those that cannot be

produced by our bodies and therefore must be supplied by the food we eat.

Nutrients are needed to ensure our bodies function efficiently.

Nutrients needed to maintain health and to give us energy are:

- ➢ **Carbohydrates**
- ➢ **Proteins**
- ➢ **Fats**
- ➢ **Vitamins & Minerals**
- ➢ **Air & Water**

Air and water are not classified as nutrients but these elements are needed for basic survival.

➢ **Carbohydrates**

Needed for energy. There are two main groups.

Simple   - found in fruit, vegetables, table sugar and milk

Complex   - found in cereals, grains, beans, potatoes & bread

➢ **Protein**

Needed for growth in babies and children.

Repairs and replaces tissues in adulthood.

Protein comes from the Greek word meaning 'of prime importance'. We need protein to enable our bodies to rebuild and repair cells (e.g. muscle tissues). A diet devoid of adequate protein leads to muscle wastage. This explains the rapid weight loss experienced on very low calorie plans. On the other hand, a diet too high in protein leads to a toxic state called ketosis. The recommendation is to eat approximately 1g protein per 1kg of body weight.

Found in meat, poultry, fish, milk, eggs, cheese, pulses, oats, nuts and soya.

> **Fats**

Needed for heat.

Protects organs from damage.

Aids in the absorptions of certain vitamins.

Found in meat, poultry, fish, eggs, dairy products, nuts and seeds.

Fat is explained in full on page 36.

> **Vitamins & Minerals**

Needed for a variety of body functions and optimum health.

Vitamins, with the exception of Vitamin D, which is produced by the action of sunlight on skin, cannot be made and have to be provided by the food we eat.

A balanced diet is needed to obtain vitamin intake.

MINERALS

Minerals are as essential as vitamins. They work with vitamins for many functions and are essential for good health. Various factors inhibit absorption of vitamins and minerals; medication, alcohol, caffeine, ill health, cooking preparation, cooking methods and exposure to light.

If you are a little confused about vitamin and mineral nutrition here is a quick reference table.

Familiarise yourself with the various roles that vitamins and minerals play and you will begin to realise that a diet rich in processed food will eventually make you ill as well as overweight.

Don't be tempted to go and buy loads of vitamin supplements. Overdoing vitamin and mineral intake can be toxic. Qualified nutritionists can identify deficiencies and the correct supplements can be prescribed.

> **Air**

Needed to breathe.

> **Water**

Water is a very important element. Many people are walking around in a dehydrated state without even recognising it.

Water is needed to help flush fat from the body but it is also needed for our bodies to survive.

We can go without food for many days but we would only last a short while without water. Try to develop the habit of drinking water at regular intervals. A slow steady stream is better for our bodies opposed to an avalanche every now and then.

ROLLS OF VITAMINS AND MINERALS

	FUNCTION	GOOD SOURCE	EFFECT OF A DEFINCIENCY
A	tissue growth, healthy skin & hair, vision, helps the body resist infection	liver, fish, eggs dairy, carrots, spinach, watercress, sweet potato, potato, mangoes, dried apricots	poor vision, dry skin, low resistance to infection
D	healthy bones & teeth, calcium & phosphorus, helps healing	oily fish & oils, fish, milk, butter & eggs	muscles & bone weakness, rickets in children
E	antioxidant, red blood cell formation, helps healing	wheatgerm, sunflower oil, sunflower seed, olive oil, nuts, eggs, green leafy veg, vegetable oils & oats, oats, avocado & wholegrain	deficiency is rare
K	clots blood to stop bleeding	green leafy veg, milk, liver, wheat bran, vegetable oils & oats	abnormal blood clotting
B1	converts food into energy, fertility, healthy heart & nervous	quorn, yeast extract, oats, pulses, nuts & seeds, meat & offal	depression, irritability, heart problems
B2	releases energy from food, healthy eyes, skin, hair, nails	yeast extract, dairy eggs, meat & offal, green leafy veg	slow wound healing, sore mouth, lips nose & problem skin
B3	releases energy from food, helps balance blood sugar, healthy skin, maintains a healthy digestive system	yeast extract, meat, fish & poultry, dairy & eggs	rare, lack of energy, depression
B5	release energy from food, helps antibodies form, healthy nervous system, healthy skin	yeast extract, liver, whole grains, avocados, eggs & nuts	rare

.	FUNCTION	GOOD SOURCE	EFFECT OF A DEFINCIENCY
B6	protein metabolism, red cell formation	yeast extract, wholemeal bread, nuts, liver, avocados, bananas, meat & fish	depression, tingling in hands and feet
B12	formation & regeneration of blood cells, energy production, healthy nervous system	meat & offal, poultry & fish, dairy & egg	anaemia, nerve troubles, vegans may suffer
FOLIC ACID	works with B12, protects against birth defects	liver, dark leafy veg, pulses, nuts & oat bran	anaemia, poor growth (nerves), depression
C	production of collagen, healing, absorption or iron antioxidant	fruit & veg, citrus, blackcurrants, strawberry, kiwi, leafy veg, peppers	dry skin, slow healing, aids muscle cramps
BIOTIN	energy production, metabolises fat & protein, healthy hair & skin, sex hormones	brewers yeast, liver, pulses & nuts, brown rice, dairy & eggs	lethargy, depression
CALCIUM	strong bones & teeth, nerve & muscle function, blood clotting, blood pressure	dairy produce, sardines & salmon, sesame seeds, almonds, green leafy veg, soya & tofu	osteoporosis, high blood pressure, heart problems, muscle & joint pain
MAGNESI-UM	needed for energy, muscle & nerve function, balances calcium, maintains bone structure	cocoa, nuts & seeds, soya beans, peas, dried fruit, oats	rare
PHOSPH-ORUS	works with calcium & magnesium, bone structure, energy production	meat & fish, dairy, nuts & seeds	muscle weakness, depression, severe case - heart attack

.	FUNCTION	GOOD SOURCE	EFFECT OF A DEFINCIENCY
SODIUM	Regulates fluid balance with potassium	processed food, cured meats, dairy	rare, salt should be kept to a minimum in diet
POTASSIUM	works with sodium to regulate fluid, normal blood pressure	fruit & veg, fish, meat & poultry, dairy	rare as stored in body, shortage shows as lethargy, confusion, fatigue
IRON	transports oxygen, strengthen s immune system, red blood cell information, energy production, optimum mental health	red meat, seafood, chicken, fish, eggs, green leafy veg, dried apricots, cocoa	anaemia, poor circulation, depression, lack of energy, lack of concentration
ZINC	immune system, healthy skin & eyes & nails, sex hormones	oysters & shellfish, red meat, chicken & offal, dairy products	white spots on nails, poor wound healing, dry flaky skin
CHLORIDE	regulates fluid balance with sodium & potassium	olives, oily fish, cheese & peanuts	rare
SULPHUR	healthy hair, skin & nails, protein synthesis, detoxification	meat, fish & poultry, offal, eggs, spinach, brussel sprouts, cheese & dried fruit	rare, a diet very low in protein
COPPER	iron & fat metabolism, heart & muscle maintenance, nervous & immune system	shellfish, offal, nuts & seeds, whole grains, soya	fairly uncommon, anaemia, poor immune system, red blood cell damage
MANGANESE	carbohydrate & fat, heart & muscle maintenance, nervous & immune system	nuts & seeds, oat bran	rare

.	FUNCTION	GOOD SOURCE	EFFECT OF A DEFINCIENCY
IODINE	regulates thyroid hormone	seafood, dairy & eggs	thyroid troubles
CHROMIUM	insulin & glucose, function, fat & protein metabolism	red meat, liver, dairy & eggs, whole grains, rye bread, oranges & apples	high blood sugar, high cholesterol
MOLYBOD-ENUM	detoxification	grains, offal, legume, dairy, spinach, cauliflower & peas	rare
FLUORIDE	strengthens bones, prevents tooth decay	water, tea, oily fish, seafood, dairy & seaweed, toothpaste!	tooth decay
SELENIUM	works with Vitamin E as an antioxidant, thyroid hormone balance	seafood, brazil nuts, liver & kidney, meat & eggs, whole grains	areas with low selenium soil levels, muscle pain and weakness

FATS; GOOD, BAD AND DOWNRIGHT UGLY!

THERE'S GOOD, BAD AND DOWNRIGHT UGLY!

The population has become so fat obsessive. Cut back on fat and you will lose weight. There have been so many 'fad' diets linked to cutting fat from your diet ranging from a few grams per day to eating no fat in a day! IMPOSSIBLE!

All fats are not created equal

FIRST, THERE IS 'BAD' FAT.

Saturated fat – usually solid at room temperature.

This type of fat is used as energy or stored as fat in the body.

'Bad' fats include; lard, animal protein, cheese, eggs and dairy products.

A diet rich in saturated fat can lead to many health problems; obesity, heart problems and high cholesterol.

Recent studies have shown that moderate intake has no significant effect on the heart but do not over do things!

'GOOD' FATS ARE SPLIT INTO TWO MAIN GROUPS.

These fats are known as unsaturated fats and are generally liquid at room temperature.

Monounsaturated   e.g. olive oil

Polyunsaturated	omega 6 – sunflower, safflower & sesame oils plus some seeds
	omega 3 - fish, fish oils, nut & seeds

Virgin hemp seed oil and flaxseed oil contain both omega 3 and omega 6 and are very good forms.

The body needs these fats for brain and nerve function, regulating the immune system, hormone balance and healthy skin and hair. These fats are essential and are used primarily for the above functions; excess will be used for energy or stored as fat.

Omega fats are extremely important fats to include in your diet as they are paramount for good health and also help the body to burn stored fat and absorb vital vitamins and minerals.

How to increase your intake of essential fats

> ➤ **Eat more oily fish**
> ➤ **Use cold pressed, unrefined vegetable oils e.g. extra virgin olive oil, groundnut, soya or sesame oil**
> ➤ **Use Udo's choice – a perfectly balance oil (Available in health food shops)**

It is not hard to include good fats within your diet. Oily fish can be eaten with salad or on toast. Sesame oil can be drizzled over a stir-fry or as a salad dressing. Most oils can be used in moderation as a nice tasty accompaniment to salad.

Nuts and seeds make a nice snack and will keep hunger at bay for ages. Nuts have many health benefits and it is a proven fact that people who eat nuts as part of their diet are less likely to suffer from heart disease.

10/12 nuts as a snack is all you need to take you to your next meal. Sprinkle a few nuts over your salad or flaked almonds on your yogurt.

Food does not have to be boring!

DOWNRIGHT UGLY

Hydrogenated fats

Trans fats

Found in highly processed foods and snacks; crisps, biscuits, cakes, margarine and chocolate snacks.

The body has great difficulty in trying to eliminate or utilise hydrogenated fats.

Butter, although a saturated fat, is easily assimilated in the body and can be used in small amounts occasionally.

Coconut is also a saturated fat but is very easy assimilated in the body. Adding coconut milk or small amounts of creamed coconut to dishes gives a superior flavour. If you eat dishes containing coconut you will find that your appetite is satisfied. Coconut oil is very popular too with amazing health benefits.

Certain olive oil spreads contain no hydrogenated fats or trans fats.

THE ROLE OF FIBRE

Fibre is a very important element in our diet. Unfortunately, the population eats well below the recommended daily intake (18g). A few years ago, fibre rich diets became very popular as fibre has the ability to keep hunger at bay. Bran and wheat bran became very popular products but over consumption is not good nutrition. Adequate fibre intake aids digestion, eliminates harmful toxins and helps to prevent many diseases; high cholesterol, diverticulitis, bowel distension and colon cancer.

Recent studies from the EPIC trial (European prospective investigation into cancer and nutrition) published in 2003, showed that among people with below average fibre intakes (which includes most of us in the UK) doubling the amount of fibre eaten could reduce the risk of developing cancer of the colon by 40%.

Another problem with insufficient fibre intake is that it leads to constipation.

WHAT IS CONSTIPATION?

Constipation is essentially food waste that could be days old, sitting around in your body for longer than it should. Waste moves slowly through the intestine leading to a build up in the bowel. The waste becomes heavier and heavier and you are carrying that around with you day after day – so it's no wonder constipation can make you feel uncomfortable, bloated and lethargic.

WHY CONSTIPATION SHOULD NOT BE IGNORED

Waste that sits in the bowel for longer than is normal can cause the bowel wall to stretch and the muscles to function less efficiently. If it happens over a prolonged period bodies can become susceptible to many ailments both minor and major.

CERTAIN CHANGES IN LIFESTYLE CAN BE VERY EFFECTIVE AT RELIEVING CONSTIPATION.

> **Eating three regular meals – skipping meals encourages over-eating later and incorrect food**

choices can be made.
- Include good sources of fibre in your diet.
- Drinking enough fluid – this will decrease the amount of time that waste spends in the body – approx 1.5 – 2 litres per day.
- Take moderate, regular exercise – this increases movements of the colon and promotes normal bowel habits.
- Eat as naturally as possible – refined 'junk' foods are not easily assimilated by our bodies.
- Limit red meat and dairy products.

THE BENEFITS OF A FIBRE-RICH DIET.

People who eat more fibre tend to:-

- Have healthier digestive systems
- Have lower rates of constipation
- Are less likely to suffer from certain diseases e.g. diverticultis
- Are often slimmer!
- Are less likely to have heart disease
- Have clearer skin

GOOD SOURCES OF FIBRE

- Oats and oat bran
- Wholemeal and wholegrain breads
- Dried apricots
- Brown rice
- Linseed
- Pulses
- Fruit and vegetables

Bran should be eaten in moderation as over consumption leads to a binding effect on vital nutrients.

Sometime in <u>severe</u> cases dietary changes are not enough.

These products will help:

Psyllium husks or Konjac fibre

When old hard matter has been cleared *"A new healthy lifestyle can begin"*.

Laxatives are gastrointestinal irritants and are not the long term answer.

METABOLISM AND DIGESTION

Your metabolism is the total of the entire calorie burning changes that occur in the body. Metabolism is the rate at which your body burns calories and is highly affected by what you eat, when you eat and the exercise you do.

THREE FACTORS CONTROL YOUR METABOLISM

1] The thermic effect of feeding (TEF). This accounts for 5-10% of the calories you burn all day. This is the energy your body uses to digest each meal, and the amount of energy spent will vary depending on the kind of food you eat.

2] The thermic effect of activity (TEA) reflects the number of calories you burn doing any physical activity from gardening or carrying groceries to jogging a mile! TEA accounts for about 20-30% calories burned each day.

3] But the most important factor controlling metabolism is your basic metabolic rate (BMR) which is the number of calories required for your body to maintain its basic functions; pumping blood, breathing, blinking your eyes, etc. BMR takes care of 60-70% of calories burned, which is why you need to actively reset your metabolism so that it will burn that fat even when you're not exercising.

Low calorie diets actually slow down your metabolism. Skipping meals (people think they are saving calories) makes your body's metabolism slow down, hence it burns fewer calories. Your blood sugar drops, causing you to eat three times more when you get your hands on food.

TO CALCULATE YOUR BMR (BASIC METABOLIC RATE) I.E. CALORIES NEEDED

As mentioned in the eating plan I do not want people to be obsessed by calories. The idea is to understand your body and listen to your body. Use this as a guide you will soon learn how much food is needed.

If you are under 31, multiply your weight by 14.7 and then add 496.

If you are over 31, multiply your weight by 8.7 and then add 829.

Note: for this you will need to calculate your weight in kilograms.

Divide pounds by 2.2 to convert.

Any extra calories you may need depends on your activity level, so:

If you are sedentary multiply BMR by 1.4.

If you are moderately active then multiply your BMR by 1.7.

If you are very active then multiply your BMR by 2.

It has been proved that eating a balanced GI diet creates an internal metabolic balance.

DIGESTION

The digestive system is responsible for processing food,

breaking it down into reusable proteins, carbohydrates, minerals, fats and other substances and introducing these into the bloodstream so that they can be used by the body.

The digestive or alimentary tract begins at the mouth, where the teeth and tongue begin the breakdown of food, aided by saliva secreted by the salivary glands. The chewed food, combined with saliva, is swallowed, carrying it in peristaltic (contractile) waves down the oesophagus to the stomach. In the stomach, the food combines with hydrochloric acid, which further assists in breaking it down. When food is thoroughly digested, the fluid remaining called chime, is passed through the pylorus sphincter to the small and large intestine. Within the long intestinal canal, the nutrients are absorbed from the chime into the bloodstream, leaving the unusable residue. The residue passes through the colon (where most of the water is absorbed into the bloodstream) and into the rectum where it is stored prior to excretion. This solid waste, called faeces, is compacted together and, upon excretion, passes through the anal canal and anus. Along the way through the digestive tract, the pancreas, spleen, liver and gall bladder all secrete enzymes, which aid in the digestive process. It is important to balance the portions of different food groups as each food group requires different conditions for digestion. When we overload our systems with food the digestion process is impaired hence indigestion and bloating. This is a good reason for eating just enough food to satisfy and also eating as naturally as possible.

PROCESSED FOOD V NATURAL

Busy lifestyles mean less time for everybody. If you can buy your weekly meals ready prepared and all you have to do is heat them, why bother preparing your own from scratch?

The answer is:

> ➢ **Unbalanced nutrition**
> ➢ **High fat intake**
> ➢ **High sugar consumption**
> ➢ **High salt consumption**
> ➢ **Ill health**
> ➢ **Lack of energy**

SALT

This hidden ingredient has an underlying effect on weight gain and causes many fatal health problems.

"But I don't put salt on my food!"

Salt is abundant in processed food; breakfast cereal, soup, frozen meals, pizza – basically anything that is processed.

A person can consume between 10-30g salt per day eating a diet rich in processed food.

The recommended daily intake is 6g!

Salt values vary in products and you may find processed food with low quantities. It would be very difficult for the modern person to totally eliminate all types of processed food from their diet.

Striking a good balance is the key.

You may not find the word salt in the nutritional information of some products although certain products are beginning to clearly label the word salt. Salt may be labelled as sodium.

Multiply the sodium g x 2.5. This will calculate the salt value.

Salt is also a problem with the diets of children. A child between the ages of 4-6 only requires 3g salt per day. A child can consume this amount of salt during breakfast!

Salt induces thirst and what better way to quench a thirst... fizzy pop, full of sugar!

If the majority of your diet comes from processed food you will be consuming either high levels of fat or high levels of sugar (abundant in low fat products) or a combination of the two coupled with a good helping of salt.

This equates to high blood pressure leading to heart problems and strokes and... WEIGHT GAIN.

Don't be fooled by clever marketing – learn to read labels.

Marilyn Glenville (1999) believes that, *"The best kept secret of weight loss and good health is to eat as naturally as possible. Natural foods are the ones your body can digest easily and use to maximum benefit. These are the foods you can burn off swiftly which means they are good suppliers of energy and don't linger in the body causing weight gain. Research by scientists worldwide is now showing that if you look after yourself you have a better chance of preventing certain degenerative illness such as heart disease, diabetes, and cancer including breast and bowel cancer."* [Reference 2]

Eating a diet rich in natural foods is good for your health but there are certain foods that are far superior to others and should be included in your diet. These foods are often referred to as super foods or bonus foods.

The SMART GI diet plan advocates the following foods to be incorporated into your regime for optimum health and also to help prevent many degenerative illnesses. Super food lists vary in different literatures but we have included the foods that everyday people are more likely to eat.

Losing weight may be your aim but an added bonus of optimum health outsmarts other weight loss diets.

The following foods have a variety of health benefits. The prime benefits have been listed.

BROCCOLI

Contains chemicals that are proven to discourage cancer.

BEETROOT

A powerful antioxidant.

Supports a healthy immune system and may reduce the risk of cancer.

CABBAGE

Reduces risk of cancer and helps lower the risk of heart disease and strokes.

CARROT

Helps to protect us from cancer (especially lung cancer).

Lowers blood cholesterol.

LETTUCE AND OTHER SALAD GREENS

The darker the leaf the better e.g. spinach.

These foods are eaten raw so they offer rich vitamin and mineral content.

Helps reduce the risk of cancer.

Reduces the risk of heart disease and strokes.

ONION

Helps reduce the risk of heart disease, stroke and cancer.

Natural antibiotic.

Antioxidant.

SWEET POTATO

Antioxidant.

Richest low fat form of vitamin E.

BLUEBERRY

Aids the body's defences.

Powerful antioxidant.

CRANBERRY

Can help in the prevention of urinary tract infections.

Supports the immune system.

ORANGES

May cut the risk of certain cancers.

Helps the immune system.

Aids in the lowering of blood cholesterol.

CHILLI

Helps in discouraging blood clots by stimulating circulation.

Natural pain reliever.

GARLIC

Best known healing food (modern research has proved this).

GINGER

Another wonderful healing food.

OATS

Reduces blood cholesterol.

A natural nerve soother – 'a feel good food'.

SUNFLOWER

Antioxidant.

Can help in preventing angina.

WALNUT

Lowers blood fats and cholesterol.

Anti-inflammatory action.

YOGHURT

Supports the immune and digestive system.

Counteracts the side-effects of certain antibiotics.

OILY FISH

Lowers the risk of heart disease and cancer.

TOMATO

Antioxidant.

May help in reducing the risk of cancer, heart disease and strokes.

BEANS & LENTILS

Can help reduce the risk of heart disease.

Regulate blood sugar levels.

PUMPKIN SEEDS

Supports immune system.

A very powerful source of zinc.

TEA

Often a topic of criticism (stimulant).

It has been found that it may reduce the risk of cancer and heart disease.

Learn to read labels

Who reads labels?

Who can be bothered?

The labels on food packaging can be very complicated if you are unsure of what you are looking for.

The first thing to look for is the ingredients list. The ingredients on a label are listed with the first ingredient having the greatest quantity within the product and the last having the least quantity.

EXAMPLES

1) CURLY FRIES (FROZEN)

Ingredients – potatoes (81%), vegetable oil, wheat flour, salt, modified potato starch, spices, garlic powder, raising agents (diphosphates, sodium bicarbonate), yeast extract.

Per 100g of product
Energy	296K cals
Protein	3.8g
Carbohydrate	32g
(of which sugars)	0.4g
Fat	17g
(of which saturates)	9g
Fibre	3.6g
Sodium	0.7g

2) SALMON STEAKS (FRESH)

Ingredients – salmon

Per 100g of product
Energy	213K cals
Protein	24g
Carbohydrate	Nil
(of which sugars)	Nil
Fat	13g
(of which saturates)	2.5g
Fibre	Nil
Sodium	0.1g

Processed food will contain many ingredients including sugars, salts, additives and E numbers.

Some countries have banned E numbers in products due to risk of illness and adverse allergic reactions.

A product that contains many E numbers is best avoided.

Sugar can be labelled as sucrose, fructose, glucose, dextrose, lactose & maltose.

Sweeteners are:
Acesulfame-K   sweeteners slow down
Aspartame   the digestive process
Saccharin   and increase appetite!
Thaumatin

Salt is listed as sodium and/or salt.

Hydrogenated vegetable oils. These are best avoided. Found in margarine, crisps, burgers, biscuits and processed food.

As a rule of thumb, a product with an extremely long ingredients list should make you suspicious about the naturalness of that product. The chances are there will be ingredients that you have not heard of. These products tend to resemble a chemistry lesson and should be well avoided.

It is quite a shocking fact that many people put these products into their shopping trolleys with no idea what is contained within them.

Manufacturers will argue that the additives, preservatives and flavourings make up a small percentage of the food. The trouble here is if we eat all processed and packaged food that percentage will be high.

In a nutshell, you will be eating food that is sadly lacking in vitamins and minerals.

If you lead a busy lifestyle it is impossible to prepare everything yourself and there will be times when you need to buy packaged food. They are not all bad; choose the ones with the smallest, most natural ingredients list.

BREAKDOWN OF NATURAL INFORMATION

CARBOHYDRATES

These are sometimes split between starch and sugars.

PROTEIN

States grams of protein in a food (this depends on size etc).

FATS

The saturated fat should be a separate figure.

FIBRE

States how much fibre per item and/or 100g.

SODIUM

States how much salt in a product.

THE SMART GI DIET PLAN

SIMPLE – MANAGEABLE – ACCURATE – REVOLUTIONARY – TESTED

SETTING A REALISTIC TARGET!

If you want to carry through a project as ambitious as reducing your own bodyweight, you need to set yourself a realistic target.

1. Determine you BMI (Body Mass Index page 5).

2. Choose an article of clothing that you would like to fit into or even an article of clothing that would look much better with a few less pounds to squeeze into it!

3. The scales (for weight) are not always the best means of ascertaining if you are overweight. Specialised scales are now available to measure fat percentage and water percentage. These are only a guide as the machines only highlight the quantity of fat and give no indication of the distribution of the fat mass in the body.

4. Before you start your new eating plan I suggest you take your measurements (table to record them is found later in this book page 207).

5. Another measurement to be aware of is your waist measurement over 35 inches 89cm for women and 37 inches 94cm for men is deemed as a risk to health.

If you have a considerable amount of weight to lose split the weight into smaller chunks. Smaller goals will lead you to your ultimate target.

Stay positive and you will succeed.

It is quite normal to lapse from time to time. Do not perceive these lapses as failure. Start again the next day and yes, you've guessed it... stay positive!

To begin a new eating regime you will need to understand the correct "tools of the trade".

> **Positive attitude**
> **Smart food choice**
> **Regularity of meal**
> **Become more active**

If you have come directly to this chapter to find out what food you can eat etc please go back and read the previous chapters.

You need to fully understand why people and diets have failed in the past.

SIMPLE GUIDELINES

> **Eat regular meals – breakfast being the most important**
> **Familiarise yourself with portion sizes and forget calorie obsession**
> **Learn satiety – eat until satisfied!**
> **Reduce stimulants (tea, coffee & canned drinks)**
> **Eat as naturally as possible**
> **Develop the habits of reading labels carefully**
> **Ensure you are eating enough fibre**
> **Essential fatty acids – make sure these are included in your daily food intake**
> **Reduce intake of saturated fat, refined sugar & salt**
> **Focus on your target at all times and stay positive**

> **If you over-indulge one day – don't give up, just get back on track the next day**

A NOTE ABOUT SATIETY

Eat until satisfied!

This does not mean eat until stuffed!

Calorie counting can be very tedious and counterproductive. Imagine you have a daily calorie quota and at some point you have to choose to go over it or go hungry.

Situations like this lead to people not eating enough food or the total opposite – a big binge!

Learning to listen to your body and finding out how much food is needed to satisfy can be very rewarding. Learn this and you will have mastered the most important tool that will get you off the yo-yo dieting treadmill forever.

Make smart food choices and your body will do the counting for you!

The secret is to trick the body into burning unwanted fat by eating enough food to maintain a steady metabolism and at the same time concentrating on reducing saturated fats and refined sugars.

If your brain does not think it is "on a diet" you are more than likely to succeed.

Guides to portion sizes have been worked out for you.

BREAKFASTS

On rising, blood sugar is at its lowest. For example, if we retire at 11pm and our last meal was at 6pm, at 8am it would be fourteen hours since we last ate. If breakfast is omitted and our first meal is at noon this would be eighteen hours! The body needs replenishing in the morning to enable it to work and function efficiently.

Breakfast should consist of slow release energy foods as this will determine how we feel for the rest of the day. Many people skip breakfast as they think they are saving calories. Your body does not understand this action and goes into a 'starvation mode' hence, the next meal will not only be stored as fat reserves it will probably be the wrong food choices and a tad bigger that normal!

BREAKFAST VARIATIONS

Popular commercial cereal contains great amounts of sugar, caramel etc. Even cereals that contain no sugar are still refined in some form or another. Low fat does not necessarily mean they are good for you! Choose cereals which are made from whole grains. These will sustain you for longer.

WHOLEGRAIN CEREALS
Oatmeal
Porridge oats
Muesli (no added sugar)
Wholegrain Rye flakes
Millet rice cereal
Oat bran cereals
Kasha breakfast pilaf
BEST OF THE REST
Quaker oat bran crispies
Eat Natural breakfast cereal
Special K
Shredded wheat
Bran flakes/All bran

Porridge can be made with skimmed or semi-slimmed milk and/or water. Some people eat it raw with cold milk! Don't get confused with instant hot oat cereal, use pure oats. Strict vegans use soya or rice milk (rice milk has been labelled as a bad food that can cause weight gain. The Chinese would not agree!). If you are dairy intolerant and really dislike soya milk, apart from water, there really isn't anything else to use. Certain rice milks are naturally flavoured with vanilla and taste delicious.

Porridge can be slightly sweetened; use a small amount of honey, all fruit jam, maple syrup or a sprinkle of brown sugar. Cereal can be eaten with hot or cold semi-skimmed or skimmed milk or low fat yoghurt.

Portion size   –   approx 6 fluid ounces milk/3tbsp milk

This can be slightly bigger depending on activity levels and climate.

Muesli   –   3-4tbsp/6fl.oz milk

Cereal   –   a cereal bowl full!

BREADS

Bread has become a popular topic of diets. There is so much conflicting advice regarding the GI and health value of breads. Let's look at this sensibly and practically.

If you have been eating bread all your life and sometimes-large amounts in one sitting, you will not be able to give it up. This plan does not advocate giving bread up for good; quality and quantity are the important factors.

Low GI/GL breads are soya and linseed, pumpernickel and German rye bread. These breads have different textures and tastes from other breads. You will either love them or hate them.

There are so many types of bread in the supermarket; white, brown, wholemeal, multi-grain, seeded, soda etc. Whole bread lacks fibre and doesn't sustain you; certain brown breads are white flour that has been dyed.

100% wholegrain bread is sometimes difficult to find and if the rest of your family won't eat it, it will be wasted. The extremely organised could freeze packs of two slices!

WHOLEGRAIN BREADS
Soya & linseed
Wholemeal stone ground
German Rye bread
100% wholegrain
Pumpernickel
Multi-grain
Granary
Soda bread

New breads arrive on the supermarket shelves all the time.

Duchy Originals (Prince Charles' organic food company) have produced a few organic loafs which are available in supermarkets.

The oat bread is absolutely delicious.

Toast is easy to make in the morning and can be eaten with an all fruit jam e.g. St Dalfour, which is available from supermarkets. Another topping idea is a little honey or even a scraping of natural peanut butter! These toppings can easily replace butter or margarine.

Other ideas for when you have more time or at the weekends for example are: -

Scrambled egg on toast

Tinned tomatoes on toast

Portion size – two slices

FRUIT

Ideal for hot days or when you have eaten too much the previous evening or the days when lunch is earlier than usual. Fruit on its own is not recommended on a regular basis as this does not fill you up. Fruit can be eaten prior to another breakfast choice or eaten with a natural low-fat yoghurt or skimmed milk product of your choice e.g. Total 0% Greek yoghurt.

FRUIT		
Apples	Apricots	Blueberries
Blackberries	Blackcurrants	Bananas
Cherries	Cantaloupe melon	Grapefruit
Galia melon	Kiwi	Lemon
Mango	Nectarines	Oranges
Peaches	Papaya	Plum
Strawberries	Other fruits	

If you are not used to eating breakfast fruit is a good choice. It is easy to eat and comes ready prepared!

Portion size   – 2/3 fruits.

Example: strawberries, blueberries with chopped banana with a small pot of yoghurt.

Fruit smoothies are becoming very popular. Whizzing fruit with yoghurt can make a simple smoothie in a liquidiser.

A FACT ABOUT FRUIT

Fruit is a very important part of our diet. It supplies our bodies with vital vitamins, minerals and fibre. Fresh fruit should be preferably on an empty stomach. If fruit is eaten directly after the other food its digestive journey will be impaired and will cause fermentation. This can be uncomfortable as it causes flatulence and bloating. If you allow the fruit to ferment in your stomach the valuable nutrition will be lost.

The exception to this is low sugar fruits i.e. berry fruits; strawberries, raspberries, blueberries etc which you can eat with other food or at the end of the meal without any problems. Also, fresh pineapple contains specific enzymes to break down protein, helping to ease digestion. You can also eat cooked fruit at the end of a meal, as cooked fruit does not ferment in the stomach. Do not forget that most of the vitamins are lost in cooking.

Eat fruit before a meal (approximately twenty minutes) or wait a couple of hours after a meal e.g. as a snack between breakfast and lunch or lunch and evening meal.

PROTEIN BREAKFAST

It is nice to occasionally treat yourself to an English cooked breakfast but be careful not to overdo it!

A nice treat at weekends as a late breakfast after a lay in!

PROTEINS	ACCOMPANIMENTS
Scrambled egg	Tomatoes (tinned)
Poached egg	Mushrooms
Omelette	Baked beans (no added sugar)
Lean bacon grilled	
Turkey bacon grilled	

Portion size   - 2 rashers lean bacon
                     - 1 poached egg

- Omelette or scrambled (1 egg/2 egg whites)
- 2 tbsp beans
- Tomatoes/mushrooms – as much as you like

Some people like kippers for breakfast!

Eat the food you enjoy.

Breakfasts can be mixed to suit each individual.

NOT TIME FOR BREAKFAST?

If you really make a mad dash to work in the morning or you start work far too early to contemplate food take a breakfast bar.

Eat Natural breakfast bars are far superior to any other bar and they taste divine. They are suitable for people with gluten intolerance (available in supermarket).

DRINKS

Make sure you drink enough fluid at breakfast. The body needs rehydrating at this time. Water with lemon juice is a good start to the day. If your are a coffee/tea addict it is recommended that you drink in moderation. Some diets insist you give up coffee and tea but that can be extremely difficult if you have drunk them all your life. Try and limit yourself to one to two cups. Decaffeinated Arabica coffee is a good choice.

SWEETENERS

The odd teaspoon of sugar in coffee is ok but try to avoid sweeteners, as they are difficult to digest and increase appetite.

Remember, breakfast is the most important meal of the day.

LUNCH

People often say *"If I eat breakfast, I am ravenous by lunchtime!"*

Depending on breakfast choice this generally means your metabolism is working. Breakfast skippers can actually feel less hungry than the people who have enjoyed a hearty breakfast.

SALAD

Salad does not have to be lettuce with a mixture of food that neither fills you up nor satisfies. On the contrary, salad should be enjoyed and can be quite easily made in a box and taken to work.

EXAMPLE:-

Lettuce, tomato, cucumber, celery, radish, onions, peppers, leftover cooked vegetables. The list is endless.

Lettuce can be as plain as iceberg or buy a mixed bag of salad leaves. Supermarkets stock every type of lettuce in these bags; rocket, spinach, radicchio, lambs lettuce etc.

CHOOSE A PROTEIN

Cooked chicken,

Cooked turkey.

Tuna, mackerel, prawns, sardines, seafood etc.

Lean ham or beef (avoid processed meat – yuk!).

Avocado pear (good fat that really fills you up).

Mixed beans (tinned or cook your own).

Hard-boiled egg.

Portion sizes:-

-   Meat, fish and poultry – approximately the size of a palm (4-6oz 110-150gm)
-   Examples:-
-   Small tin of sardines, 185g tine of tuna, one chicken breast
-   Avocado – half
-   1 hard boiled egg
-   3 tbsp mixed beans

You can keep it simple or add a small sprinkling of seed.

Dress with olive oil/white wine vinegar and lemon juice or a dash of Newman's own salad dressing (made from an original recipe from Paul Newman).

Eat as much salad that fills you up.

SOUP

Soup is a wonderful filling food. Either make your own or buy a good natural alternative (for people who have no time) e.g. Baxter's, Covent Garden – available at all supermarkets.

To make your own simply chop any combination of vegetables or a single vegetable, boil and simmer with stock (vegetable bouillon is a good choice), add herbs and spices and a dash of Worchester sauce. Add meat if desired (leftover cooked meat). Eat as a chunky soup or blend in a liquidiser. Soup can be taken to work in a food flask or if you have microwave/hob facilities it can be heated and eaten quickly and easily.

Eat with a slice of wholegrain bread or a couple of oatcakes.

SANDWHICHES

The sandwich is probably the most popular lunch of all time!

Think quantity and quality.

If you have had toast for breakfast, omit bread at lunchtime.

Sandwiches are easy to make and easy to eat.

Choose bread from the breakfast list or use wholemeal pitta bread or tortilla wraps and fill with a protein (look at salad list) add salad.

Other ideas for lunch are houmous (dip made from chickpeas) with raw vegetables and oatcakes.

Jacket potato with protein (try sweet potatoes).

Omelette.

LUNCH ON THE RUN

There will be times when you need to buy your lunch e.g. when you are out for the day or when the fridge is empty!

Shops are full of pre-packed sandwiches and salads. Go for multi grain bread with a salad and protein filling (no mayonnaise) or choose a salad bowl that looks fresh without a fatty dressing.

Skipping lunch is not a good idea. If you are a lunch skipper, what do you do when you arrive home? Eat? Look at what you eat and be honest with yourself. Is it normally food that is quick to eat, highly processed and full of fat. Why? Because you let your body get over-hungry.

EVENING MEALS

Eating something in the evening is more likely to cause

weight gain than eating something in the morning or at lunchtime! The body builds up its reserves again during the night.

If you starve your body of fuel (food) during the day it goes into a metabolic conservation mode. Look at it this way, you've put it through your everyday routine devoid of fuel.

"I haven't eaten much today, so I can have a real feast when I get home tonight!"

A real feast can turn into: raiding the cupboard and fridge, eating whilst preparing the meal and then snacking all night long.

If this is continued, weight loss will be practically impossible and metabolism will become so slow that the metabolic fire will burn inefficiently.

If possible, the evening meal should not be too heavy. If you are feeling very hungry, not enough food has been eaten throughout the day.

As a guide it should consist of:

> **Lean protein**
> **Small portion of starchy carbohydrates (if desired)**
> **Good portion of vegetables**

Protein   = size of palm (4-6oz/110-150g)
Carbs   = the same
Vegetables = unlimited

The combination of foods balances the overall glycaemic load.

1) CHOOSE A PROTEIN

Fish is a wonderful low-fat protein with many health benefits.

Fish should be bought fresh and a good fresh fish bares no smell.

Fish contains fat that is a 'good fat'; omega 3 and this is very good for you. A food that is good for you does not mean that it will still be good for you if deep-fried in batter or breadcrumbs! Even if you remove the outer covering a good proportion of the fat it has been fried in will have accumulated within the fish.

Fish cooks very quickly and can be steamed, poached, grilled or baked in the oven. Add lemon juice and herbs prior to cooking and you will have a wonderful low-fat, nutritious protein.

People who eat more fish tend to be much healthier, have better digestive systems and live a longer life.

FISH			
Cod	Coley	Crab meat	Cockles
Herring	Haddock	Halibut	Lobster
Mackerel	Monkfish	Mussels	Oysters
Prawns	Sardines	Salmon	Swordfish
Squid	Sole	Sea Bass	Tuna
Other fish		There are many varieties	

MEAT

Choosing the best cuts of meat begins when we purchase it.

I would recommend that you choose a good butcher who concentrates on buying and preparing good quality meat. Ask a good butcher where he sources his meat and he will quite confidently tell you the whole history of the meat you are purchasing.

Always buy lean cuts of meat where possible. Visible fat can be trimmed prior to cooking.

It is recommended by The Royal College of Physicians that no more than 5oz/140g of red meat should be eaten in one day.

This equates to the portion size = size of palm.

Beef   – choose leanest cuts.
Lamb   – choose leanest cuts.
Pork   – choose leanest cuts.

Red meat is not totally banned but be careful not to over consume.

Poultry & Game

POULTRY	GAME
Chicken (no skin)	Hare
Duck (no skin)	Partridge
Goose	Pheasant
Ostrich	Rabbit
Turkey	Venison
Quail	

Chicken and turkey are very low-fat proteins.

Most people would choose these two options from the above table as they are versatile and very easy to purchase and cook.

VEGETABLE PROTEIN

You don't have to be a vegetarian to enjoy these proteins. It is nice to have a meat free day occasionally. Many people are unsure of how to cook vegetable proteins or what to add to them for taste. See Recipes on page 156.

VEGETABLE PROTEIN
Dried beans (soaked & boiled)
Chickpeas
Lentils
Quorn
soya

2) CHOOSE A CARBOHYDRATE

A small portion of carbohydrate is all that is needed at the end of the day. If you decide to exercise after work the portion can be larger to replenish energy stores.

Remember, carbohydrates are required for energy. Eating a large serving at your evening meal prior to settling down to a night in front of the television will only encourage your body to store the excess.

Portion sixe = size of a palm.

POTATOES

Potatoes have become a popular subject on their role in weight gain. The potato is a nutritious vegetable and needs to be eaten as nature intended. A new potato will contain less starch than an old one and is the better choice. The trouble comes when the potato is refined, processed and turned into various snacks; crisps, chips and instant mash. Jacket potatoes are an easy meal once in a while but choose your filling wisely! We associate jacket potatoes with melted butter and usually, large amounts! If the thought of eating a potato without lashings of butter makes you cringe, avoid them. It is important that you eat the foods you enjoy. Try baking sweet potatoes.

Other carbohydrate choices are brown basmati rice or plain brown rice.

Portion size = approximately 3 tbsp.

Egg noodle - these come in packets of four squares.

Portion size – 1 square.

Wholemeal pasta (Al dente – which means just cooked approx 6 minutes) or whole with spaghetti.

Portion size – approximately 3 tbsp.

There are other whole grains that can be tried e.g. Quinoa. Very similar taste to rice and cooked in the same way.

Or couscous, which is very easy to prepare.

Eat the foods that you enjoy.

3) VEGETABLES

Vegetables, like fruit are natures own vitamin supplements.

They can be steamed, stir-fried, lightly boiled, microwaved or eaten raw.

Fill your plate up with a variety of seasonal vegetables and enjoy.

Accompaniments and flavour enhancers.

Season food with herbs and spices. There are so many different flavours to be explored. Season-all (Schwartz), mixed herbs, Worcester sauce and bay leaves are a basic set for any kitchen.

PUDDINGS

Sample ideas.

Natural yoghurt with summer fruits.

Cooked fruit.

Plain chocolate (70% cocoa) in moderation as a treat.

Home-made ice-cream.

Frozen yoghurt dessert.

SNACKS

There are various reasons for snacking.

Maybe you are hungry?

Maybe you are bored?

Maybe you skipped a meal?

Having the correct choice of snacks to hand is the key.

Fruit.

Yoghurt.

A few nuts (10-12 almonds as an example).

Oatcakes.

2/3 dried apricots.

BEVERAGES

Drink 6-8 glasses fresh water each day.

Water with lemon juice.

Tomato juice.

V8 vegetable juice.

Pure apple juice.

Decaffeinated coffee (1-2 cups ordinary coffee is ok).

Tea (1-2 cups).

Herbal tea.

Fruit tea.

Many people are walking round in a dehydrated state and don't even realise it. If you complain about headaches on a regular basis, this could be one reason for them,

Alcohol.

The recommendation for alcohol is to have a maximum of 5 units per week. A unit is one glass of wine, ½ pint beer or lager or one measure of a spirit.

HAVING A TREAT DAY

Set the alarm for 6am. Get up and eat all day long! No!

Having a day off is about going out and eating something you enjoy without feeling guilty about doing it.

If you are going out for an evening meal don't starve yourself all day. Eat normal meals and then you will not need to eat half the menu of buffet when you get there.

Meeting friends for a cappuccino at the week-end? Have a cappuccino and enjoy it, you don't do it every day!

MAKING WISE FOOD CHOICES

In an ideal world, we would all grow our own vegetables, purchase organic meat and produce and prepare everything from scratch. Unfortunately, life is not as simple as that. Every day we learn that vegetables contain pesticides, meat contains hormones and fish have toxins from the water they live in.

It is all about making the wisest choices possible. Buying everything organic is far too expensive to the everyday, working person and why shouldn't we trust food manufacturers? They must follow guidelines? Certain foods will get better and others will get worse. As a general guide, buy fresh food regularly rather than keeping it stored for days on end in a fridge or a fruit bowl. Purchase meat, fish and poultry that look as fresh as possible.

SAUCES AND GRAVY

People tell me all the time that they cannot possibly eat food without gravy or sauces.

A little gravy on a dinner is much better than a plate full of burger and chips covered in tomato sauce. Always read the labels on cooking sauces.

You will find recipes for tasty sauces on page 180.

GI is a proven science. If the word science conjures up a diet full of complicated calculations – don't worry.

Making a few simple changes to your existing diet may be all that is needed to adopt a low GI diet.

- ➤ **Change your normal breakfast cereal to a whole grain. Porridge or natural muesli**
- ➤ **Choose grainy breads opposed to white or brown. These are breads that contain seeds, oats and multi grains.**
- ➤ **Incorporate pulses and legumes (pearl barley, chick peas, lentils etc) into your diet by adding them to soups and salads.**
- ➤ **Eat adequate fibre e.g. dried apricots as a snack**
- ➤ **Try to eat at least one low GI food with every meal. Eating low GI foods with high GI foods makes the overall GI of a meal – moderate.**

Experiment with foods to find the ones you enjoy.

Make small changes gradually and you will find that your new way of eating becomes 'a way of life' and not a 2 week wonder diet!

2 WEEK SAMPLE MEAL PLAN

Use this as a guide, mix and match as you wish.

DAY ONE

Breakfast	Porridge with semi-skimmed or skimmed milk or water
Mid-morning	Fruit
Lunch	Chicken salad sandwich made with wholegrain bread
Mid-afternoon	Fruit/yoghurt
Evening meal	Fish with vegetables and rice

DAY TWO

Breakfast	2 slices wholegrain toast with all fruit jam
Mid-morning	Fruit
Lunch	Large salad with tuna
Mid-afternoon	10 almonds/2 dried apricots
Evening meal	Chicken stir-fry (unlimited vegetable) with brown basmati rice

DAY THREE

Breakfast	Quaker oat-bran crispies with semi-skimmed or skimmed milk
Mid-morning	Fruit
Lunch	Chunky vegetable soup with pearl barley, slice of bread
Mid-afternoon	Fruit/yoghurt
Evening meal	Spaghetti bolognaise

DAY FOUR

Breakfast	Poached egg on wholegrain toast
Mid-morning	Fruit
Lunch	Chicken salad with houmous dip
Mid-afternoon	Fruit

| Evening meal | Prawn & cashew stir-fry with roasted Mediterranean vegetables. |

DAY FIVE

Breakfast	Porridge with semi-skimmed or skimmed milk
Mid-morning	Fruit
Lunch	Chicken & Vegetables soup with pasta shapes
Mid-afternoon	Fruit & nuts
Evening meal	lentil Curry (Dahl)

DAY SIX

Breakfast	Special K with semi-skimmed or skimmed milk
Mid-morning	Fruit
Lunch	Salad with mixed beans
Mid-afternoon	Yoghurt
Evening meal	Salmon steaks with green vegetables & brown rice

DAY SEVEN

You could have a day off here and have a treat day or have a similar plan from above. It's up to you!

DAY EIGHT

Breakfast	Grilled bacon with mushroom & tomatoes
Mid-morning	Fruit
Lunch	Chunky vegetable soup with wholegrain bread
Mid-afternoon	Fruit
Evening meal	Chicken, vegetables & boiled new potatoes

DAY NINE

Breakfast	Fruit with natural yoghurt
	Banana, blueberries, strawberries
Mid-morning	handful of mixed nuts
Lunch	soya & linseed bread sandwich (protein of your choice with unlimited salad)
Mid-afternoon	Fruit
Evening meal	Braised steak with vegetables

DAY TEN

Breakfast	Porridge with semi-skimmed or skimmed milk
Mid-morning	Fruit
Lunch	Salad with sardines
Mid-afternoon	Fruit
Evening meal	Chicken with tomato, onion & garlic with vegetables

DAY ELEVEN

Breakfast	Wholegrain toast with baked beans
Mid-morning	Fruit
Lunch	Prawn salad
Mid-afternoon	Fruit/yoghurt
Evening meal	White fish in parsley sauce with unlimited vegetables

DAY TWELVE

Breakfast	Quaker oat-bran crispies
Mid-morning	Fruit
Lunch	Wholegrain sandwich with protein of your choice and salad
Mid-afternoon	Fruit
Evening meal	Turkey breast with new potatoes & vegetables

DAY THIRTEEN

Breakfast	Eat Natural cereal bar
Mid-morning	Fruit
Lunch	Wholemeal pitta filled with protein of your choice and salad
Mid-afternoon	Fruit/nuts
Evening meal	Thai green chicken curry with brown basmati rice

DAY FOURTEEN

It's treat time again!!!!!!!!!!!!

Use the portion sizes listed in the plan as a guide and enjoy your food.

Getting the balance right is the key for weight loss and also for good health. Eating red meat every day may upset the digestion system and overdo saturated fat consumption; once or twice a week is probably enough. Experiment with vegetable proteins and different types of fish.

The important thing to remember is to enjoy your food. Eating something you really don't like just because it is good for you is a recipe for failure.

Keep a food diary for your own records.

A food diary can be useful to identify problem times during a day or even identifying certain trigger foods i.e. foods that trigger a sweet raid for example!

COOKING METHODS & UNTENSILS

It is really a good idea to make your own meals.

Cooking does not have to be time consuming, a little preparation, the correct tools and easy cooking methods may change your mind about cooking.

You may even enjoy it!

HEALTHY COOKWARE

It is a good idea to invest in a good quality set of saucepans; stainless steel, glass or cast iron. These will last for many years and there is no risk of linings contaminating your foods.

Non-stick pans are OK but if the base shows any signs of scratching or peeling – get rid.

A basic kitchen should have:-

- ➢ **A good set of saucepans (various sizes)**
- ➢ **A wok or large frying pan for stir-fries**
- ➢ **Wooden utensils – to avoid scratching**
- ➢ **Baking trays**
- ➢ **Ovenproof casserole dishes**
- ➢ **An electric or gas oven**
- ➢ **Hygienic chopping board**
- ➢ **Set of clean, sharp knives**
- ➢ **Tin opener**
- ➢ **Garlic crusher**
- ➢ **Colander**
- ➢ **Measuring jug**
- ➢ **Set of measuring spoons (teaspoon, dessertspoon, tablespoon)**
- ➢ **Draining spoon**
- ➢ **Mixing bowls**
- ➢ **Casserole dishes**

Other useful gadgets are:-

> ➢ **Microwave oven**
> ➢ **Steamer**
> ➢ **Slow cooker**
> ➢ **Food processor**
> ➢ **Liquidiser or blender**
> ➢ **Health grill**

There are so many gadgets nowadays but if you have everything from the list (basic kitchen) you will not go far wrong.

GUIDELINES FOR COOKING

BEST OILS AND HOW TO STORE THEM

Always purchase oil in a glass, preferably dark glass bottle. Oils, when exposed to heat, light and air tend to turn rancid more quickly. Keep oils in a cool dark place and always airtight.

Buy a bottle a month (which should be enough) and then replace with a new one. There are so many oils to choose from in the supermarkets, olive oil is a good all rounder. It can be heated to a hot temperature and also used as a salad dressing cold.

Certain oils are not recommended for hot temperature cooking e.g. wok cooking.

VEGETABLE COOKING

Vegetables can be steamed, boiled, microwaved, roasted and stir-fried.

Vegetables lose their nutrient content from the moment they are cut from the ground and then deteriorate more when prepared.

Peel and chop vegetables just before you need them to obtain optimum vitamin and mineral content.

STEAMING

Either in a steamer or over a pan of boiling water with a fan steamer (round metal plate with holes that can be adjusted to fit various saucepans).

MICROWAVING

Vegetables are placed in a casserole dish (with lid) and micro waved in a very small amount of water. Modern micro wave ovens have a vegetable sensor button. Just press vegetables and it works out how long it needs and then pings when ready!

BOILING

The old fashioned way. Well, they didn't have any other methods years ago. The nutrients are lost in the water.

STIR FRYING

Quick and healthy in a wok.

ROASTING

Vegetables are placed on a baking tray, drizzled with olive oil and roasted in a hot oven.

CHOOSING VEGETABLES

You can buy almost any vegetable at the supermarket. Certain people may prefer to buy vegetables from the market, farm shops or have an organic box delivered to their door.

Buy fresh vegetables as you need them.

MEAT, FISH AND POULTRY

Available in supermarkets, butchers, farm shops, fishmongers and mail order.

Meat, fish and poultry freeze quite well so a monthly visit to the butcher would save time. There are companies that will deliver fresh meat to your door.

There are many different cooking methods, which will be explored in the recipe section (page 86).

GRAINS AND PULSES

Porridge oats and other grains e.g. brown rice can be stored in an airtight container and keep well for a few weeks.

Pulses are a very low fat protein. They can lower cholesterol, help to control diabetes and are a valuable low GI ingredient in a weight loss plan.

Pulses need to be introduced in the diet slowly as an overload leads to uncomfortable flatulence.

They can be purchased as a dry pulse which needs to be soaked prior to cooking or they can be found ready to use in a can (easy!).

Soaking and cooking instructions should be clearly labelled on packaging. As a general rule of thumb, the larger the pulse – the longer it needs to be in soak.

Soaking overnight is the best option.

FLOUR

You may find plans recommending that you convert to soya flour or use ground almonds in place of flour. If you are prepared to experiment with these flours all well and good but if you only need the odd ounce of cornflour to make a sauce (which makes a very nice basic white sauce) or to thicken a casserole etc stick to what you know. Yorkshire pudding made with substitute flour may taste a little weird, let alone become very expensive! The odd Yorkshire pudding made with your Sunday dinner will not sabotage your good work. Yorkshire pudding made with substitute flour is no longer Yorkshire pudding! Yorkshire people would be truly horrified. Pastry, doughnuts and other fast food that is rich in white flour, sugar and fat is the real problem here and that is what you need to severely cut back.

HERBS AND SPICES

All supermarkets now stock herbs and spices in various forms; fresh, dried powders, dried flakes and ready chopped with oil in jars and tubes. You can even buy a growing pot for the kitchen windowsill!

A basic stock for the cupboard

- ➢ **Ground black pepper in a pepper mill**
- ➢ **Ready mixed curry powder**
- ➢ **Ready mixed chilli powder**
- ➢ **Schwartz season-all**
- ➢ **Dried mixed herbs**

Fresh herbs can be purchased weekly (approximately 50p for a small bag or carton). The adventurous gardener could grow their own.

It is well worth experimenting with herbs as they give food a unique flavour and have many health giving properties.

RECIPE IDEAS

You will find various recipe ideas for breakfast, lunches, evening meals, snacks and puddings.

We have included some very basic recipes and also a few ideas for the more adventurous.

You will be able to find all the ingredients in supermarkets.

BREAKFASTS

- ➢ **Cereal**
- ➢ **Breads**
- ➢ **Fruit**
- ➢ **Protein**

LUNCHES

- ➢ **To take to work**
- ➢ **To enjoy at home**

EVENING MEALS

- ➢ **Meat**
- ➢ **Poultry**
- ➢ **Fish**
- ➢ **Vegetarian**

Kim G Bryan

BREAKFASTS

Kim G Bryan

PORRIDGE

Porridge can be made in the microwave or on the hob in a pan.

How you cook porridge depends on the consistency required.

MICROWAVE METHODS

You will find various methods on the back of oats packets.

Either mix the milk and oats together and microwave the mixture at 30 second intervals (stirring after 30 seconds).

Or

Heat the milk first in a microwaveable bowl – approximately 1 minute. Add the oats and then microwave the mixture at 30 second intervals until you get the consistency you require.

STOVE TOP METHOD

Place oats in a saucepan and add either cold water, milk or a combination of the two. Bring to boil and simmer for 2-3 minutes, stirring occasionally.

Porridge can be sweetened with all fruit jam, honey, maple syrup or a sprinkle of Demerara sugar.

A little sweetness added to porridge will not undo the goodness of this staple breakfast.

Check the portion sizes on page 58.

SMART MUESLI

This can be made in bulk and stored in a container for daily use.

Porridge oats
Rye flakes
Golden linseed
Sunflower & Pumpkin seeds (optional)
Small portion or mixed chopped nuts (almonds, walnuts etc)
Chopped dried apricots
Small portion desiccated coconut (optional)

Mix all ingredients together and eat with a milk of your choice (from breakfast list page 59) hot or cold.

The oats and rye flakes should make up the bulk of the muesli and the other ingredients should be added in smaller quantities.

For people with gluten intolerance - gluten free oats can be purchased and rice flakes can be substituted for rye flakes.

JENNY'S GRANOLA

700g rolled oats
50g pecans (break into pieces)
50g slivered almonds
200g sunflower seeds
100g linseed (brown or golden)
100g sesame seeds
Mix together in a large bowl.

Mix up
3 tbsp olive oil (or sunflower)
3 tbsp liquid honey
1 tbsp black treacle
250ml warm water

Add to the dry mixture and stir in. (I also add 2 tbsp fig jam as they grow in my garden.)

Spread the mixture out onto a baking sheet (it takes about 3 of my baking trays).

Bake at 180'C for about ½ hr.

When it's cool add dried fruit, cranberries, apple, mango, cherries, pineapple, apricots, strawberries etc.

I usually use about 250g of assorted dried fruit, but adjust for your taste.

Store in airtight containers.

Enough for 2 people for about 3 weeks (makes a good crumble topping).

LEN'S BRAN & BERRIES

2-4 tbsp bran flakes
Handful of raspberries
Handful of strawberries
Handful of blueberries

Mix the bran flakes with the berries.

Eat alone or with milk.

Yoghurt or any other skimmed milk product e.g. low fat fromage frais can be used in place of milk.

EASY FRUIT SMOOTHIES

In a blender or smoothie maker.

Whizz natural yoghurt with a fruit of your choice. You can substitute milk yoghurt for soya yoghurt.

Good choices are:-

> - Strawberries
> - Banana
> - Kiwi
> - Blueberries
> - Raspberries

Experiment with different combinations. If you prefer to make the smoothie as a drink, add a little skimmed milk to the mixture. A little honey, maple syrup or fructose (fruit sugar) can be added if desired. Sprinkle with a few flaked almonds.

Smoothies are an excellent way of introducing children to a healthy breakfast. You can be as inventive as you wish. Add a tablespoon of muesli or add natural breakfast cereal to the mixture and blend with the ingredients.

Drink as a drink or serve in a cereal bowl and eat with a spoon.

If you suffer with milk allergy - use soya yoghurt.

GRILLED RUBY RED GRAPEFRUIT

One ruby red grapefruit.

Sprinkle of Demerara (optional).

Slice the grapefruit in half.

Sprinkle with a small amount of sugar on each half and grill for approximately 2 minutes.

This breakfast can be eaten prior to another choice as it will not keep you going all morning!

A nice start to a Sunday morning prior to a mid morning brunch.

SUNSHINE BREAKFAST

Make a cereal bowl full of:-

- ➢ Strawberries
- ➢ Banana
- ➢ Kiwi
- ➢ Blueberries
- ➢ Raspberries

Squeeze a little lemon juice over the fruit.

Eat alone or with low-fat natural yoghurt (total 0% Greek yoghurt).

Top with a sprinkling of flaked almonds if desired.

Add a teaspoon of runny honey or maple syrup.

SOYA AND LINSEED TOASTIES

Burgen soya and linseed bread or choose another grainy bread.

Toast 2 slices of soya and linseed bread.

Add a topping of your choice:-

> ➢ All fruit jam
> ➢ Natural peanut butter
> ➢ Tinned tomatoes
> ➢ Scrambled or poached egg
> ➢ Cheese! One of my clients swears by this breakfast!
> ➢ Grilled lean bacon with tomatoes
> ➢ Kippers!

You will not need to add butter or margarine.

THE HEALTHY ENGLISH BREAKFAST!

It is nice to occasionally treat yourself to an English breakfast.

Ideal as a late Sunday breakfast.

Lean bacon
Tinned tomatoes
Mushrooms
Poached egg

Bacon can be grilled or cooked on a health grill.

Mushrooms can be steam fried in a little oil and water to soften.

Use a fry pan or wok with a lid.

Sausages?

Certain sausages from butchers are full of meat and others contain little meat and loads of fat.

If you possess a health grill most of the fat can be eradicated.

Go for a sausage that contains quality meat (usually purchased from a good butcher) not one that is bright pink!

Kim G Bryan

LUNCHES

- SALADS -

SUNSHINE SALAD

Serves 1

Leafy salad greens
Cherry tomatoes – halved
Red pepper – sliced
Yellow pepper – sliced
Orange pepper – sliced
Grated carrot
1 tbsp sunflower seeds

Combine all salad ingredients together either on a plate or a salad box for work.

Serve with:

HONEY AND MUSTARD DRESSING

1 tbsp unrefined sunflower oil
150ml/¼ pint low fat natural yoghurt
Juice of 1 lemon
1 tsp wholegrain mustard
1 tsp honey
Ground black pepper

Combine all ingredients in a bowl and stir well. Season to taste.

The amounts in this can serve up to four people but the dressing can be stored in a fridge for up to three days.

AVOCADO AND WATERCRESS SALAD

Serves 2

Watercress
Iceberg lettuce leaves
Chopped cucumber
Chopped celery
1 avocado
Chopped spring onion
Lemon juice

Make a lettuce bed with the iceberg and watercress.

Add the chopped cucumber, celery and spring onion.

Slice the avocado and drizzle with lemon juice.

Serve alone or with:

YOGHURT AND MINT DRESSING

1 tsp fresh chopped mint
1 tsp fresh chopped parsley
1 tsp fresh chives

Liquidise with a little natural yoghurt to make a puree.

In a bowl, stir in 200ml/7fluid ounces natural yoghurt, juice of ½ lemon and ½ tsp paprika. Stir well. Season with black pepper.

SALMON SALAD WITH PINEAPPLE SALSA

Serves 2

2 salmon steaks (cooked) or large tin of red salmon drained.
Salad vegetables of your choice; leaf, cucumber, tomato etc.

PINEAPPLE SALSA

100g/3½oz finely chopped fresh pineapple.
1 red pepper finely chopped
1 tsp green chilli, deseeded and finely chopped
Handful of fresh coriander – chopped – approx 3 tsp
1 tbsp lemon juice

Combine all ingredients in a bowl and stand for ten minutes. Substitute the salmon for another oily fish. Change the lemon juice to lime or combine both lemon and lime for a totally different flavour.

NOTE: if you suffer when chopping fresh chillis, substitute the chillis for dried chilli flakes.

The salsa can be stored in the refrigerator for two days.

Alternatively, if salsa is not for your taste buds, substitute for another dressing or use Newman's Own (available at supermarkets).

WALDORF SALAD

Serves 2

2 red apples
4 celery stalks chopped
25g/1oz roughly chopped walnuts
Chopped fresh herbs to garnish
Squeeze of lemon

Wash apples and dry.

Dice apples and combine with lemon juice in a bowl.

Add celery and walnuts.

DRESSING

1 tbsp walnut oil (can be substituted for another oil)
Juice of lemon or orange
Ground black pepper
150ml/¼ pint low fat natural yoghurt

Combine all ingredients together.

Add dressing to salad ingredients and garnish with herbs.

Note: this salad and dressing will not store.

PRAWN SALAD WITH TOMATO SALSA

Serves 2

8oz/225g fresh or frozen (defrosted) prawns
Salad green
Choice of salad vegetables

TOMATO SALSA

250g/9oz tomatoes
3 spring onions finely chopped
1 green chilli, deseeded and finely chopped
2 tbsp lemon or lime juice
Fresh coriander

Peel tomatoes.

Score the skin and cover with boiling water for two minutes, lift out with a fork and the skin should come off easily.

Chop the tomatoes and combine with the remaining ingredients. Leave for twenty minutes.

Do not store.

The tomatoes can be substituted for other ingredients e.g. peppers.

To add an extra bite to salsas add some crushed garlic!

TUNA NICOISE SALAD

Serves 2-3

A large handful of iceberg lettuce
or mixed salad leaves
8 cherry tomatoes – halved
½ cucumber – sliced
1 red onion – sliced
2 hard boiled eggs – sliced
Handful of pitted black olives
1 large tin of tuna in spring water or brine or 2 freshly cooked
tuna steaks
Squeeze of lemon

DRESSING

4 tbsp extra virgin olive oil
1 tbsp white wine vinegar
1 peeled and crushed garlic clove
Ground black pepper and 1 tsp sugar

Place all the salad ingredients in a bowl and mix with the
lemon juice.

For the dressing:-

Whisk the oil, vinegar, garlic and pepper in a bowl until
combined.

Place the mixed salad vegetables onto each plate. Add the
tuna to the centre of the salad vegetables. Scatter the hard-
boiled egg slices and olives over the salad. Spoon the
dressing over the salad. Garnish with parsley.

CHICKEN SALAD

WITH MEDITERRANEAN VEGETABLES AND BALSAMIC DRESSING

Serves 2

3-4 tbsp Mediterranean vegetables – hot and cold
The recipe for this can be found on page 161.
2 average chicken breasts – sliced
Salad leaves e.g. iceberg, spinach, radicchio etc.
8 cherry tomatoes
½ cucumber sliced

Serve above as a mixed salad

BALSAMIC DRESSING

2 tbsp extra virgin olive oil
1 tbsp balsamic vinegar
1 tsp wholegrain mustard
1 tsp sugar

Mix all the ingredients together well.

Or use:-

Newman's own balsamic dressing (available at supermarkets).

CRUNCHY SALAD

120g/4oz washed and diced carrots
60g/2oz celery sliced
Red pepper – diced
45g/1½oz chopped walnuts
2 tbsp sweetcorn
½ tsp paprika
Pinch of chilli powder
2 tbsp Newman's own French dressing

Place carrots, celery, pepper, sweetcorn and walnuts in a bowl.

Mix the paprika and chilli into the French dressing and pour over the ingredients.

Chill for 30 minutes.

Serve this salad as a side salad or add chicken breasts to eat as a main meal or lunch.

COLD MEAT PLATTER WITH NEW POTATOES

Salad leaf
Cucumber
Tomatoes
Spring onions
Red onions
Cooked beetroot – sliced
(allow 3-4 per person)

mixture of cold meats
lean ham, cooked chicken,
cooked turkey
choose lean cuts of meat
allow 2 slices (average)
per person

Cook the new potatoes in boiling water with fresh mint leaves until soft. Approximately 10-15 minutes (test with skewer).

Arrange the salad vegetables.

Serve with meat, potatoes and cooked beetroot.

Salads can be taken to work in an airtight container.

Add the dressing just before eating.

Salads can be eaten as an evening meal if desired.

- SOUPS -

STOKES SOUP KITCHEN

Mrs. Dorothy Stokes, a distinguished lady who grew up during the war, offers practical advice about preparing, making and storing soup.

Homemade soup really takes no time at all. The question is can we be bothered!?

Dorothy says, *"If you feel in the mood for soup making, it is a good idea to make bulk amounts and freeze into portions."*

She also added, modern equipment i.e. blenders and food processors have decreased the preparation time of vegetables. We no longer have to cut everything into tiny pieces as the blenders do it all for you!

As for ingredients, anything goes! Experimenting with different vegetables can be very rewarding. It all depends whether you like to taste the vegetable or prefer a more seasoned soup.

If you do not possess a blender, don't worry. Chunky soups are just as tasty

WINTER VEGETABLE CHUNKY SOUP

Chop a variety of vegetables into bite size chunks.

- ➢ Carrot
- ➢ Celery
- ➢ Swede
- ➢ Parsnip
- ➢ Potato
- ➢ Sweet potato
- ➢ Leeks
- ➢ onions

The quantity depends on whether you are making a soup for one or a bulk amount.

Mix vegetable stock. Vegetable bouillon powder is a good choice as you can mix just enough for one without wasting any.

If you really want a tasty soup, boil a chicken carcass in water to make real chicken stock.

Boil until all the chicken has fallem off the bones. Discard bones. Boil the vegetables in whatever stock you choose and then simmer until tender. Season with black pepper. Red lentils or pearl barley can be added to this soup at the vegetable stage to make a bulkier, more filling soup.

CARROT AND CORIANDER SOUP

550g/1lb carrots
1 tsp extra virgin olive oil
1 tsp butter
1 pint vegetable stock
2 tsp fresh chopped coriander
Ground black pepper
Soured cream to garnish (optional)

Wash and peel carrots and cut into chunks.

In a large saucepan:-

Heat the oil and butter. Cook the carrot chunks gently for two minutes
Add the stock and bring to the boil.
Cover the pan and reduce the heat.
Simmer for fifteen minutes.

In a blender or food processor:-

Liquidise the carrot mixture with the fresh coriander. Season.

Swirl soured cream to serve – if desired.

Variations can be made with different vegetables and herbs.

Using the same recipe and method, substitute carrot and coriander for:- fennel with lemon thyme, broccoli with onion, celeriac with parsley – experiment with your own.

QUICK AND EASY
VEGETABLE AND
CHICKPEA SOUP

Serves 2

50g/1¾oz chickpeas (cooked)
500ml/7½fl.oz stock
50g/1¾oz peas (fresh or frozen)
1 large chopped onion
1 tbsp fresh chopped coriander
Ground black pepper

In a saucepan:-

Heat the stock.

Add the peas and simmer for two minutes.

Add the remaining ingredients and heat for two minutes.

Serve.

FRENCH ONION SOUP

Serves 2

2 onions
30g/1oz butter
15g/½oz cornflour or soya flour
490ml/7 fluid ounces vegetable stock (hot)
Ground black pepper
Grated cheese to garnish (optional)

Cut onion into rings
Sauté in a pan with the butter until browned.
Mix the flour in until browned.
Gradually add the stock, stirring all the time.
Add ground black pepper.
Simmer for thirty minutes.

Serve in soup bowl and sprinkle a little grated cheese on the top.

A note from Dorothy:

To thicken a soup, add a few chunks of potato.

A handful of pasta shells is another idea at lunchtime. Add to the soup prior to cooking. Almost, anything goes in a soup!

If you have any leftover cooked meat this can be added near the end of the cooking.

Ensure the meat is thoroughly reheated.

MINESTRONE
A MEAL IN ITSELF!

4 rashers lean bacon
1 large onion – chopped
2 cloves garlic – crushed
2 sticks of celery – finely chopped
½ swede, finely sliced
1 courgette, diced
2 potatoes, diced
1 tsp fried mixed herbs
1 can chopped tomatoes
1.75 litres/3 pints stock
50g/2oz dried whole-wheat spaghetti broken into small pieces
½ savoy cabbage, finely shredded
300g can borlotti beans, drained
50g/2oz grated parmesan cheese

Heat a little oil in a pan. Add the bacon, onions and garlic and fry for about five minutes. Add the remaining vegetables apart from the cabbage and beans. Add the herbs, canned tomatoes and stock.

Bring to the boil and then cover the pan and gently simmer for about an hour ensuring all the vegetables are cooked.

Add the spaghetti pieces, shredded cabbage and beans and cook for a further ten minutes. Sprinkle in half the cheese, season to taste and add extra stock if needed.

Sprinkle the remainder of the cheese prior to serving.

The vegetables can be varied according to what you have available or what is in season.

SANDWICHES-

Kim G Bryan

PITTA BREAD WITH HOUMOUS AND SALAD

Serves 2

2 wholemeal pitta breads
Slice iceberg lettuce
1 red onion sliced
2 tomatoes sliced
¼ cucumber sliced

QUICK HOUMOUS – IDEAL AS A SPREAD OR USE A DIP

200g/7oz drained chickpeas (canned or cooked)
100ml/3½ fluid ounces tahini paste
2 crushed garlic cloves
1 tsp ground cumin (optional)
4 tbsp lemon juice
2 tbsp extra virgin olive oil
1 tsp paprika

Place all ingredients into a food processor or blender and whiz to a puree. Coarse or creamy depending on personal preference.

Add more liquids if needed. Add paprika.

Split the pitta breads and spread the houmous onto each side. Fill the split pitta with the salad ingredients.

AVOCADO & SARDINES ON GRAINY BREAD

Serves 2

4 slices good quality bread (choose from bread list in breakfasts page 59)
1 avocado (ripe)
1 tin sardines
2 cherry tomatoes finely sliced
Squeeze of lemon juice

Cut the avocado in half and remove the stone.
Scoop out the flesh.
Spread over the slices of bread. Add a squeeze of lemon.
Open the sardines and drain.
Place equal amounts of sardines on the bread with avocado.
Place the sliced cherry tomatoes on top.

Eat as an open sandwich or as a sandwich.

Substitute the sardines for another protein.

Sandwiches are probably the most popular lunch of all time but we don't need to eat them every day! Choose good quality fillings. Avoid processed meat and heaps of mayonnaise and you will succeed.

- EGGS -

EGGS ARE A VERSATILE FOOD

They can be:-

> Soft boiled
> - boil for approximately 3 minutes (size dependant)
> Hard boiled
> -boil for ten minutes
> Poached
> - In a poaching pan or the old fashioned way. Bring a small saucepan full of water to the boil and add two or three splashes of vinegar. Drop the broken egg into simmering water and cook to preferred consistency – approximately two minutes.
> - eggs can be microwaved in a ramekin dish – one minute
> Scrambled
> - beat eggs and heat gently in a saucepan. Add a little milk if desired.
> - microwave on a high power, stirring every thirty seconds
> Fried! – occasionally as a treat!
> - crack the egg into a frying pan and don't be tempted to add loads of oil!
> Omelette
> - basic omelette

2 eggs
A little milk
1 tsp water

Beat all the ingredients together. Add the mixture to an omelette pan or frying pan. Heat gently until eggs have set.

OMELETTE VARIATIONS

Almost anything can go into an omelette.

> ➤ Mushroom and onion
> ➤ Chopped lean bacon with tomato
> ➤ A small amount of grated cheese
> ➤ Leftovers!

Scrambled egg is another versatile dish with eggs.

Scrambled egg can be flavoured with mustard, which gives this dish a unique flavour.

The guidelines for egg consumption changes all the time. As a guide, eat up to four per week.

Kim G Bryan

AN EASY TEN-MINUTE OMELETTE MEAL

Serves 1

Basic omelette mix (as on page 126)

Handful chopped mushroom
1 rasher lean bacon – chopped
1 small onion – chopped
A little extra virgin olive oil to sauté

In a frying pan, heat the oil. Add the onions, heat until soft – approximately 2 minutes.

Add the bacon and mushrooms and heat for a further two minutes.

Add the omelette mixture over the top of the onion, bacon and mushrooms. Make sure the egg mixture covers the whole of the frying pan. Heat gently for 2-3 minutes.

Meanwhile, pre-heat the grill.

Ensure the omelette is cooked underneath (should resemble a light golden brown colour).

Place the pan under the grill and grill the omelette for approximately 3 minutes. This finishes the cooking of the eggs and makes a bulkier omelette.

-EVENING MEALS-

EVENING MEALS

Most people will have set ideas about the food they eat. Some of us prefer meat and vegetables without any fancy flavouring whilst other are prepared to experiment a little in the kitchen.

You will find a few ideas for:-

> ➢ Chicken
> ➢ Meat
> ➢ Fish
> ➢ Pulses

You will also find a few vegetable accompaniments.

If you enjoy cooking it is well worth experimenting with a few ideas of your own.

Remember, food does not have to be boring!

Marinating tenderises meat, fish and poultry and provides excellent flavours.

Marinate for at least 1 hour or even better, overnight.

COOKING MEAT IN A SLOW COOKER

Not time to cook? Invest in a slow cooker and your dinner will be ready when you get home!

If you are a bit worried about leaving appliances on whilst you are out make a large quantity on a day off and freeze portions.

EASY CHICKEN

Place the whole chicken in the slow cooker prior to leaving for work and leave to cook.

The chicken will make its own juices.

The cooked chicken can be eaten that night with vegetables or carve the chicken for later use.

EXAMPLES:-

> Cold meat platter
> Add to soup
> Add to vegetable curry

COOKING JOINTS

Add water to nearly cover the joint. Add vegetables to the water e.g. onions, carrot, leeks, swede etc.

Slow cookers can be used for casseroles, curries and soups. Most slow cookers come with an easy recipe guide.

COOKING IN A WOK

Wok cooking is quick and easy. A meal in minutes.

Wok cooking is best carried out on gas hobs, as it is easier to control the heat.

Basically, anything goes in a stir-fry recipe. Dishes can be either cooked in a sauce or slightly glazed with a flavour.

E.g. sweet and sour chicken (cooked in a sauce) or meat and vegetables with a dash of soy sauce or honey. Mince is also easy to cook in a wok.

CHICKEN
WITH TOMATOES,
ONION AND GARLIC

Serves 2

2 chicken breasts – sliced or chunked
Tin of chopped tomatoes
2 crushed garlic cloves
1 large onion chopped
Ground black pepper & 1 tsp season all
Dash of Worcester sauce

In a wok:-

Heat a little oil and add the onions and garlic. Heat until soft.

Add the chicken and stir-fry for five minutes. Ensuring the chicken is sealed.

Add the tomatoes, black pepper, season-all and dash of Worcester sauce.

Cook for approximately ten minutes.

Serve with brown basmati or egg noodles.

CHICKEN AND CASHEW NUT STIR FRY

Serves 2

2 chicken breasts – sliced
1 courgette – sliced
1 red pepper – sliced
1 chopped onion
2 crushed garlic cloves
2 tsp lemon grass
Handful of cashew nuts
1 tbsp soy sauce

In a wok:-

Heat a little oil. Add onions, garlic & lemongrass. Cook until soft. Add the chicken. Cook and seal.

Add the peppers and cashew nuts. Stir-fry quickly for 3-4 minutes. Add the courgettes and soy sauce. Stir fry for a further 2 minutes.

Add a little water and place the lid on the wok. This will steam fry the vegetables and cook them quicker. Serve with brown basmati rice.

Other vegetables can be used in stir-fries:-

> Mange-tout
> Baby sweetcorn
> Green beans

Use the vegetables you enjoy the most. Be imaginative!

CHICKEN BREASTS
STUFFED WITH WALNUTS, ORANGE & PARSLEY

4 skinless chicken breasts
1 onion, finely chopped
2 tbsp extra virgin olive oil
50g/2oz chopped walnuts
Rind and juice of 1 orange
2 tbsp chopped parsley
1 tbsp cranberry sauce (optional)
Beaten egg mix
Ground black pepper
1 tbsp Dijon mustard

Make a slit in the chicken breasts to form a pocket. Heat 1 tablespoon of the oil and fry the onion until soft, place in a bowl to cool. Add the walnuts, orange rind, parsley, cranberry sauce and enough beaten egg to bind together

Divide the cooled stuffing mixture between the chicken breasts pushing it into the pockets. Spread the Dijon mustard over the chicken breasts with the seasoning and place in an ovenproof dish. Drizzle over the remaining oil and juice from the orange.

Place in a pre-heated oven 190c/375f/gas 5 for 25 minutes. Baste a couple of times during cooking.

Serve hot with seasonal vegetables or cold and sliced with a salad.

CHICKEN WITH LIME AND THYME

Serves 4

4 chicken quarters or chicken breasts (without skin)
Lime juice to cover chicken
¾ pint chicken stock
1 bay leaf
2 tbsp chopped parsley
1 tsp chopped thyme
225g/8oz brown rice

SAUCE

1 medium sliced onion
2 medium tomatoes – chopped
2 tsp mustard

Marinate the chicken in the lime juice for one hour. Drain off marinade.

In a large saucepan, place the chicken and stock. Bring to the boil and simmer for approximately one hour (depending on the size of the chicken). Drain off the stock and put to one side. Add the bay leaf, parsley, thyme and rice to the stock, make the stock up to 1½ pints with more water. Add the chicken pieces back to the stock and cook for approximately thirty minutes.

Meanwhile, heat a little oil in a frying pan and sauté the chopped onions until brown. Add the chopped tomatoes and mustard. Cook on low heat until cooked. Mix the sauce into the chicken and rice mixture. Remove bay leaf. Serve with a selection of green vegetables.

GREEN THAI CURRY

Serves 2

2 chicken breasts – sliced or cubed
1 chopped onion
2 crushed garlic cloves
2 heaped tsp Bart Thai Green curry paste
(other brands are available at supermarkets)
1 tsp Bart lemon grass or 1 tsp freshly chopped lemon grass.
(available as a fresh herb at most supermarkets)
Dash of Blue dragon fish sauce
Green vegetable e.g. handful of chopped fine green beans
1 sliced courgette or 1 chopped leek
2 lime leaves
1 can coconut milk

In a wok:-

Heat a little oil. Add chopped onion, garlic and green Thai curry paste. Add a little water and fry for approximately 2 minutes.

Add the chicken to the mixture and cook for 5 minutes ensuring that the chicken is thoroughly sealed.

Add the coconut milk and lime leaves. Simmer for 25-30 minutes. Add the green vegetable and cook for a further 5 minutes. Serve with brown basmati rice and a side salad.

Substitute the chicken for 8oz prawns, 10oz tofu or a mixture of green vegetables.

-QUICK AND EASY-
BEAN AND CHICKEN STEW

1 can of beans (cannellini, black-eyed, borlotti etc)
1 large onion
1 crushed garlic clove
1 tin of tomatoes
1 tbsp chopped fresh parsley
2 cooked chicken breasts – chopped into chunks
200ml/7¼ fluid ounces stock

In a saucepan:-

Soften the onion and garlic in a little oil for 2 minutes.

Stir in the remaining ingredients and simmer for 3-4 minutes.

Serve.

Any leftover meat can be used in this recipe; beef, lean ham etc.

CHICKEN CASSEROLE

Serves 2

2 chicken breasts
¾ pint chicken stock
1 carrot – chopped
1 large onion – chopped
22.5g/8oz button mushrooms
1 tsp season-all

In a casserole:-

Add the chicken, stock, vegetables and seasoning.

Cook in a moderate oven 180c/350f/gas 4 for 1½ hours.

After 1 hour of cooking, mix 1 tsp of cornflour with a little water and stir into the casserole to thicken.

This recipe would work well in a slow cooker.

Substitute the chicken stock for red wine to make coq au vin.

The alcohol evaporates during cooking but the wine still adds a wonderful flavour.

ROAST GARLIC CHICKEN

1 whole chicken
A whole garlic bulb
½ lemon

Preheat the oven to 180c/250f/gas 4.

Place the lemon inside the chicken.

Separate the cloves from the garlic bulb and peel.

Place the cloves all around the chicken – crush some garlic cloves and spread the garlic over the chicken.

Place in a roasting dish and cover with foil.

Cook, depending on size of chicken, 20 minutes per 1lb plus 20 minutes extra.

The chicken will make its own juices. Baste occasionally.

Serve with vegetables or carve for later use e.g. cold meat.

SHONA'S QUICK CHILLI

Serves 4

450g/1lb lean mince
1 large onion – chopped
2 crushed garlic cloves
Chilli powder – quantity depends on desired heat.
1 tin red kidney beans
1 can chopped tomatoes

In a wok:-

Heat a little oil. Add onion and garlic. Heat until soft.

Add mince. Stir the mince to ensure all mince is thoroughly sealed.

Add the tomatoes, beans and chilli powder.

Simmer for approximately 30 minutes.

Vegetarians can substitute mince for soya mince or quorn mince.

Serve with brown basmati rice and green side salad.

CHEATS CHILLI!

Serves 3-4

500g/1lb lean mince
1 large onion
1 crushed garlic clove
1 tin mixed beans in tomato sauce
Chilli powder to desired heat

In a wok:-

Heat a little oil. Add onions and garlic. Cook until soft.

Brown the mince.

Add the tinned beans and chilli powder.

Simmer for 30 minutes.

Serve.

BOLOGNAISE MINCE

Serves 3-4

500g/1lb lean mince
1 large onion
1 crushed garlic clove
1 tin chopped tomatoes
2 tbsp tomato puree
2 handfuls of chopped mushrooms
Green and red pepper, diced
1 tsp season-all
2 tsp dried mixed herbs or:-
2 tsp freshly chopped basil and oregano

In a wok:-

Heat a little oil. Add onions and garlic. Heat until soft. Add the peppers and heat for a further 2 minutes.

Add the mince and cook until thoroughly sealed. Add the tinned tomatoes, tomato puree, season-all and herbs. Add the mushrooms into the mixture. Simmer for 30 minutes.

Serve with whole-wheat spaghetti.

Alternatively, add a dash of Worcester sauce in place of the herbs for a totally different flavour.

Bolognaise and chilli recipes can be cooked very easily in a slow cooker.

Brown the mince slightly and add all the ingredients to the slow cooker.

BEEF CASSEROLE

Serves 2-3

10oz/280g stewing steak
1 large onion chopped
2 carrots – sliced
1 small potato diced
225g/8oz button mushrooms
1 pint stock
1 tsp conflour mixed with a little water to thicken (added at the end).

Add all ingredients to a casserole and stir well.

In a moderate oven – 180c/350f/gas 4 cook the casserole for approximately 1½ hours.

Add the cornflour near the end of the cooking time.

This casserole can be quite easily cooked in a slow cooker.

GERMAN MUSTARD BEEF

Good quality joint of beef e.g. topside.

1 jar German mustard.

Preheat oven to 180c/350f/gas 4.

Place the beef in a roasting dish and smother with German mustard.

Wrap joint in foil and cook slowly – allow 20 minutes per 1lb/500g plus an extra 20 minutes.

Cooking time will vary depending on whether you prefer a well-done joint or one that is still slightly red in the middle.

Serve with seasonal vegetables.

This beef can be eaten cold. E.g. cold meat platter.

STUFFED PEPPERS

Serves 2-3

Use the recipe for bolognaise or chilli.

3 large peppers – any colour.

Cut the stalk end off the pepper and keep.

Scoop out the seeds and insides of the peppers.

Fill the peppers with the cooked mince mixture and replace the ends.

Line a baking dish with foil and place the peppers upright.

If the peppers won't stand up easily – make a little tray with foil to help them.

Brush the peppers with a little olive oil.

Roast in a moderate oven 180c/350f/gas 4 for 30-35 minutes.

LIVER, ONION AND VEGETABLE CASSEROLE

Serves 2

200g/7oz liver – lambs, pigs or ox
1 large onion – sliced
1 carrot - sliced
1 leek – sliced
8oz/200g mushrooms
¾ pint stock

Place all the ingredients in a casserole dish and stir well.

Cook the casserole for 1½ hours in a moderate oven 180c/350f/gas 4.

Add a little cornflour mix towards the end to thicken, if needed.

Kidney can be added to this casserole or alternatively use pork tenderloins.

A good old-fashioned recipe - cooking like it used to be!

Serve with new potatoes and vegetables.

FISH

WHAT TO DO WITH FISH!

Fish can be:-

- ➢ Steamed
  -the healthiest way, use a steamer
- ➢ Microwaved
  -ready in minutes!
- ➢ Grilled
  -grill both sides. Easiest method to add more flavour
- ➢ Baked in the oven
  -poached in a sauce or just cooked plainly
- ➢ Stir-fried
  -ideal method for seafood e.g. prawns

Fish is a wonderful, health giving, low-fat protein.

It can be plain i.e. no sauces added. People who like the taste of fish may prefer to eat it this way.

Cooked in a sauce as basic as parsley sauce or cooked with exotic flavours.

The easiest method for a quick meal is in a microwave.

Modern microwaves have a button especially for fish. The oven works it all out for you!

Fish takes approximately 15-20 minutes to cook in an oven depending on size.

Be careful not to overcook the fish as this makes the fish rubbery!

COD IN PARSLEY SAUCE

Serves 2

2 average fillets of cod
15g/½oz cornflour
15g/½oz butter
½ pint semi-skimmed milk
2 tbsp chopped fresh parsley

Wrap the fish in foil and cook in a moderate oven 180c/350f/gas 4.

Add a little lemon juice to the parcels.

In a small saucepan:-

Melt the butter. Stir in the cornflour. Allow to bubble. The mixture should resemble honeycomb.

Stir in a little milk at a time and stir briskly, working the mixture into the milk.

Replace on the hob and heat gently, stirring all the time. Bring to the boil and simmer.

The mixture will gradually thicken.

Add the parsley and cook for a further 5 minutes.

Pour the sauce over the cod and serve with new potatoes and green vegetables.

GRILLED FISH
WITH A LEMON AND MUSTARD DRESSING

5 tbsp extra virgin olive oil
2 tbsp lemon juice
1 tsp Dijon mustard
Ground black pepper

Place all ingredients in a small saucepan.

Heat slowly for two minutes, stirring all the time.

Pour over grilled fish of your choice.

Thin fish e.g. sea bass, trout, lemon sole – 3-5 minutes.

Thicker fish e.g. cod, swordfish – 8-10 minutes.

Salmon – 6-8 minutes.

Variations of this dressing are:-

Substitute the Dijon mustard for:-

> ➢ 3 tbsp chopped tomatoes (tinned or fresh)
> ➢ Finely chopped fresh herbs; parsley, thyme or dill

EASY SALMON

Serves 2

2 salmon steaks
1 tbsp extra virgin olive oil
1 tbsp lemon juice
Chopped dill sprigs

Preheat oven to 180c/350f/gas 4.

Cut two separate squares with tin foil.

Place each salmon steak onto a tin foil square.

Add equal amounts of olive oil and lemon juice to each steak.

Place the chopped dill on each steak.

Fold the tin foil around each steak to make a parcel.

Place in a baking dish and cook for 15-20 minutes.

Serve with new potatoes and green vegetables.

STIR-FRIED PRAWNS
WITH HONEY AND LIME

Serves 2

225g/8oz fresh or frozen (defrosted) prawns
4 tbsp lime juice
Handful of mange-tout
Handful of baby sweetcorn (sold as a pack in supermarkets)
Handful of fine green beans
1 tbsp honey

Marinate prawns in lime juice for at least one hour.

In a wok:-

Heat a little oil. Add mange-tout, sweetcorn and beans. Stir-fry quickly for 2-3 minutes.

Add prawns and stir-fry for a further 2 minutes.

Add honey and stir well, coating all the ingredients.

Serve with rice and side salad.

MARINATED COD
WITH STIR-FRIED VEGETABLES

Serves 2

2 average cod fillets
Juice of 1 lime
1 tbsp extra virgin olive oil
Pinch chilli flakes
Coriander sprigs

Mix the rind, juice, oil and chilli flakes together.

Place the cod fillets in a shallow dish. Rub the marinade over the fillets. Cover and marinate for 30 minutes.

Grill the fish under a medium grill for approximately 3 minutes each side, ensuring the fish is thoroughly cooked.

Stir-fried vegetables:-

4 spring onions
1 red chilli, deseeded and finely chopped
125g/4oz mushrooms (shiitake – good choice)
225g/8oz roughly chopped bok choy
2 garlic cloves, peeled and chopped
125g/4oz carrots cut into fine batons
1 tbsp sesame oil
2 tbsp soy sauce

In a wok:- heat the oil. Add spring onions, mushrooms, garlic, carrots and chilli. Stir-fry for 2 minutes. Add the bok choy and stir-fry for a further 2 minutes. Add the soy and stir-fry for 1 minute. Serve the fish with the stir-fried vegetables. Garnish with coriander.

STIR-FRIED SEAFOOD
WITH GARLIC, LEMON AND PARSLEY

Serves 2

225g/8oz ready to eat seafood (prawns, muscles, cockles, squid rings etc, seafood selection is available as a mixed pack in supermarkets, fresh or frozen). You can use prawns alone if desired.

2 finely chopped garlic cloves
2 tbsp extra virgin olive oil
Rind and juice of 1 small lemon
2 tbsp chopped fresh parsley
Ground black pepper
Parsley leaves to garnish

In a wok:-

Heat oil. Add chopped garlic and cook until golden. Add seafood and stir-fry quickly. Drain the juices and keep.

In a separate saucepan:-

Place the reserved juice from the seafood with the lemon rind and lemon juice.

Bring to the boil and cook for 4 minutes. The sauce should thicken slightly (syrupy).

Add the seafood mixture to the hot sauce, add the parsley and re-heat gently.

Season and serve. Garnish with parsley.

-VEGETARIAN DISHES-

AND VEGETABLE ACCOMPANIMENTS

VEGETARIAN DISHES

You do not have to be a vegetarian to enjoy these dishes!

You will find a few ideas for pulses and some mouth-watering curry recipes. These recipes are very easy to do and many will freeze for up to 3 months.

Remember, to soak dry pulses (red lentils need no soaking).

If you would like to try soya, tofu or quorn. Substitute any meat in a recipe and replace with one of these vegetable proteins.

Vegetables accompaniments

Vegetables are very good for you but sometimes they can be labelled as boring!

You already know you can steam, boil or stir-fry vegetables.

Adding a few extra ingredients need not be too time consuming and can make all the difference to taste and presentation.

Whether a main dish or an accompaniment, experiment a little with vegetables and you may be pleasantly surprised!

CHICK PEA CURRY

Serves 2

1 can of chickpeas (drained)
4 tbsp total 0% Greek yoghurt
50g/2oz creamed coconut or ¼ can of coconut milk
1 chopped pepper (any colour)
1 onion, chopped
2 crushed garlic cloves
¼ tsp medium curry powder
1.4 tsp chilli powder
1-½ tbsp sultanas or dried apricots, chopped
Ground black pepper

In a saucepan:-

Heat the yoghurt and coconut over a gentle heat for approximately 5 minutes.

Add the remaining ingredients and stir well.

Add a small amount of hot water if mixture appears too dry.

Simmer for 10 minute.

LENTIL DIP

Small tin of lentils
1 onion, chopped
2 crushed garlic cloves
2 tbsp extra virgin olive oil
½ tsp cumin seeds
Fresh chopped coriander
Ground black pepper

In a saucepan:-

Heat oil, add onions, garlic and cumin seeds. Cook until soft.

Add lentils and cook for 3 minutes.

Transfer ingredients to a blender or liquidiser, add coriander and blend.

This dip can be spread onto toasted wholegrain bread or oat cakes or served with salad.

LENTIL DAHL

250g/90z rinsed and drained red lentils
(Red lentils need no soaking)
600ml/1 pint water
1 chopped onion
1 tin tomatoes
½ tsp turmeric   ⇦ **(use curry powder**
3cm/1½" sliced fresh ginger   ⇦ **instead of these 3**
1tsp cumin seeds   ⇦ **for easiness)**
2 garlic cloves, crushed
Chopped fresh coriander to garnish

In a saucepan:-

Bring the lentils, turmeric (or curry powder) to the boil.

Add the onions and garlic and simmer for 20-25 minutes (lentils should be tender).

Add remaining ingredients and simmer for a further 20-25 minutes.

Stirring occasionally, add more water if needed.

BRAISED
MEDITERRANEAN
VEGETABLES WITH BEANS

Serves 2

2 tbsp extra virgin olive oil
1 chopped onion
1 red pepper, chopped
8 cherry tomatoes or tinned tomatoes
2 stalks chopped celery
2 courgettes, chopped
2 crushed garlic cloves
400g/14oz can butter beans (or use other beans)
½ tsp chilli powder or crushed flakes
1 tsp fresh rosemary (½ tsp dried)
125ml/4fl.oz water
Fresh chopped herbs to garnish

In a saucepan:-

Heat oil; add onion, celery and garlic. Cook for 5 minutes until soft.

Add rosemary, chilli and remaining vegetables and water (substitute other vegetables if desired; aubergine, leeks, carrots etc).

Cook slowly for 30 minutes (until soft).

Stir in beans and heat for five minutes.

Garnish with herbs, add ground pepper and drizzle with a little olive oil.

MUSHROOM CURRY

225g/8oz mushrooms – cut into quarters
120g/4oz finely sliced leeks
1 chopped onion
1 crushed garlic clove
3cm/1-½" chopped ginger
1 tsp curry powder (desired heat!)
1 tsp lemon juice
60g/2oz creamed coconut grated
Oil to sauté

In a wok:-

Gently fry onions, garlic, leeks, ginger and spices until soft.

Add mushrooms and a little water, cook on a low heat until soft.

Add grated coconut – add water if mixture appears too dry.

Stir in lemon juice.

Serve with brown basmati rice and a side salad.

EASY VEGETABLE CURRY
FREEZES WELL

460g/1lb mixed chopped vegetables e.g. mushrooms, cauliflower, sweet potato, carrots, fennel, okra etc.
225g/8oz chopped onions
2 crushed garlic cloves
2 tbsp extra virgin olive oil
240ml/¼ pint semi-skimmed or skimmed milk
1 tbsp white wine vinegar
1 tin chopped tomatoes
2 tsp tomato puree
1 tsp brown sugar
½ tsp vegetables bouillon
Curry powder – amount according to taste

Sauté onions and garlic until soft.

Stir in curry powder, mix well and cook for 3 minutes.

Add milk and vinegar, stir.

Add tinned tomatoes, tomato puree, sugar and stock.

Boil and simmer for 1 hour.

Add vegetables and cook until tender. Approximately 30 minutes.

Cashew nuts and sultanas can be added to this curry if desired.

WENDY'S RATATOUILLE

1 chopped onion
3 chopped garlic cloves
3 chopped mixed peppers
4 sliced courgettes
1 tin of tomatoes
2 tsp tomato puree
1 jar of passata (there are varieties flavoured with herbs in supermarkets)

In a saucepan:-

Heat a little oil. Add onions and garlic. Fry for 2 minutes.

Add the tinned tomatoes and vegetables. Heat for 2 minutes.

Add the passata and simmer for approximately 20-30 minutes.

Garnish with mozzarella.

Serve with wholegrain pasta or rice.

Other vegetables can be used e.g. celery, carrot and aubergine.

Ratatouille can be turned into a meat dish by adding chopped grilled lean bacon.

It also goes well with chicken.

ROASTED MEDITERRANEAN VEGETABLES

2 chopped onions
4 chopped garlic cloves
1 red pepper – sliced
1 yellow pepper – sliced
1 green pepper – sliced
1 slice courgette
Button mushrooms – halved
8 cherry tomatoes
 Olive oil to drizzle
Ground black pepper

Preheat oven to 200c/400f/gas 6.

Place vegetables evenly on a flat baking tray.

Drizzle with olive oil and add ground black pepper.

Cook for 25-30 minutes.

Mediterranean vegetables can be served hot with various dishes or cold with salads.

LEEKS PROVENCALE

Serves 2

3 leeks
1 crushed garlic clove
1 tin tomatoes or 2 large tomatoes chopped
1 chopped onion
2 tbsp dry white wine
1 tbsp chopped fresh parsley
Ground black pepper
Little oil to sauté

Wash, trim and cut leeks into 5 cm/2" pieces.

Boil, steam or microwave until tender.

In a small saucepan:-

Sauté onion and garlic until soft.

Stir in tomatoes.

Add herbs and wine.

Simmer for 10 minutes.

Drain leeks well and pour the sauce over to serve.

Add a little grated cheese to the top and grill for a few minutes.

KALAMATA
–CAULIFLOWER AND OLIVES–

1 cauliflower – cut into florets
2 tbsp extra virgin olive oil
1 onion – cut into rings
1 crushed garlic clove
75ml/4fl.oz water
2 tsp lemon juice
1 ½ tbsp tomato puree
Ground black pepper
8 pitted black olives
Chopped parsley to garnish

Sauté the onion and garlic until soft.

Add water and lemon juice.

Bring to the boil. Add cauliflower and cook until tender – approximately 15-20 minutes.

Remove cauliflower from liquid and place on a serving dish.

Add tomato puree to liquid and boil. Add olive and pour the sauce over the cauliflower florets.

Garnish with parsley.

Note: if you don't like olives the dish tastes just as nice without them. Don't tell the Greeks!

SWEET POTATO MASH

Serves 2

2 large sweet potatoes
Ground black pepper
25g/1oz butter
Chopped thyme (optional)

Peel the potatoes deeply to expose the orange flesh (simply scraping may make a stringy consistency!).

Boil the potatoes until very tender – approximately 20 minutes.

Mash the potatoes well. Add butter and pepper and mix well.

Stir in the chopped thyme.

Sweet potato mash can be mashed with other vegetables e.g. swede.

SWEET POTATO CHIPS!

Peel and cut into 1cm/½" square chips. Blot dry.

In a large frying pan or wok. Heat 1-2 tbsp olive oil or rapeseed oil.

Stir-fry until just tender – approximately 8 minutes.

Or:

Bake them in their jackets.

Either in an oven as you would jacket potatoes or in the microwave (combination microwave ovens make jacket potatoes very easy!).

ROAST ONIONS

Serves 2

2 large onions
Oil to brush
¼ pint vegetable stock

Preheat the oven to 180c/350f/gas 4.

Remove the roots from the onions but leave the skin.

Place the onions in a baking dish and brush with oil.

Pour the stock around the onions.

Bake for 1½- 2 hours, basting occasionally.

Cut a cross in the top of each onion.

Peel back skin and serve (the skin will peel away very easily).

MINTY PEAS WITH A DIFFERENCE

Serves 2-3

½lb frozen peas
½ cucumber
4 spring onions – trimmed and sliced
1/8 –pint half-fat crème fraiche
2 tbsp chopped fresh mint
25g/1oz butter
Ground black pepper
Pinch of sugar

Place peas in a pan and boil. Cook for 3-4 minutes.

Meanwhile, halve the cucumber lengthways, scrape out the seeds and slice thickly.

Heat the butter in a frying pan and add the spring onions and cucumber. Sauté gently for 3 minutes.

Add crème fraiche and boil for 2-3 minutes.

Add the peas, mint, sugar and black pepper.

WHO HATES THEIR GREENS?

Serves 2

450/1lb curly kale or any other cabbage
15g/½oz butter
3 rashers lean bacon – cut into strips

Boil or steam the curly kale. Drain and lay out on kitchen paper to dry.

Melt butter in a wok; add bacon and fry gently for 4 minutes.

Add curly kale and stir-fry for approximately 3 minutes until thoroughly heated.

Any green vegetable can be used for this recipe; broccoli, green beans etc.

BAKED TOMATOES

Serves 2

2 beefsteak tomatoes (smaller ones can be used)
1 crushed garlic clove
2 tsp extra virgin olive oil
2 tsp chopped fresh parsley and chives
Ground black pepper

Preheat oven to 225c/435f/gas 7.

Slice across the bottom of each tomato approximately 1cm from the bottom.

On a greased baking sheet place the tomatoes cut side up.

Score the cut side of the tomato several times diagonally.

Mix the crushed garlic with 1 tsp of oil and stir in the chopped herbs and pepper.

Spread the mixture over the tomatoes.

Replace the sliced lid on each tomato and drizzle with oil.

Bake at the top of the oven for 20-35 minutes.

Tomatoes should be soft.

Adjust cooking time if you are using smaller tomatoes.

BROCCOLI WITH GARLIC

Serves 2

220g/½lb broccoli florets
1 tbsp extra virgin olive oil
1 sliced garlic clove
Pinch chilli flakes (optional)
1 tsp lemon juice
Ground black pepper

In a wok or large frying pan:-

Heat the oil. Add the garlic and chilli flakes.

Heat until the garlic turns golden.

Add broccoli florets and stir-fry until tender.

Add lemon juice and ground black pepper.

Alternative vegetables:- cabbage, spring greens, bok choy.

-SIDE SALADS-

TOMATO AND ONION SALAD

Serves 2

2 large chopped tomatoes
4 spring onions – chopped
1 red onion – cut into rings
Ground black pepper

Combine all the above ingredients in a bowl.

Whisk 1 tbsp olive oil with 1 tsp balsamic vinegar, add a pinch of sugar.

Add to salad mixture and toss.

GREEN SIDE SALAD

Handful of spinach
Handful of lamb's lettuce
½ cucumber – sliced
2 spring onions – chopped (include all the green part)
1 green pepper - diced

Mix all the greens together and drizzle with lemon juice.

Side salads make a refreshing accompaniment to hotter dishes.

Mix and match salad ingredients to create your own.

-SIMPLE SAUCES-

SOMETIMES, ALL A MEALS NEEDS IS A SAUCE!

SIMPLE TOMATO AND GARLIC SAUCE

1 tin chopped tomatoes
2 tbsp tomato puree
3 crushed garlic cloves
2 tbsp olive oil
Ground black pepper

In a saucepan:-

Add tomatoes, tomato puree, garlic and oil. Bring to the boil.

Adjust heat and simmer for 30 minutes. Add black pepper.

Use this sauce with chicken, vegetables or pasta.

Add basil or other fresh herbs to make a herby tomato sauce.

MUSHROOM SAUCE

15g/½oz butter
A drop of olive oil
1 tbsp cornflour
½ pint milk
225g/8oz chopped mushrooms

Heat butter and oil. Sauté mushrooms for a few minutes. Remove mushrooms and set aside. Stir in the cornflour to the butter and oil. Add milk and whisk together. Bring the sauce to the boil, stirring continuously. The sauce should begin to thicken. Add the mushrooms and heat gently. For a sauce with a bite, add 1 tsp English mustard. Serve with meat, vegetables or pasta.

A basic white sauce is:-

15g/½oz butter
15g/½oz cornflour
½ pint milk

This will make ½ pint sauce. Adjust quantities for larger amounts

Anything can be added to this sauce e.g. cheese, mustard, parsley, onion etc.

Sauces can make the most boring of vegetables taste delicious and they take no time at all.

Kim G Bryan

-PUDDINGS!-

Maybe you have rushed to this page to see what is in and what is out of bounds in the pudding category!

Well, good news and bad news!

If you say to yourself *"I will never be able to eat another pudding if I am going to get this weight off!"*

You are kidding yourself and you will inevitably fail.

From time to time occasions will arise when you are faced with the ever-tempting sweet trolley!

It is nice to go out and the last thing you need is to say *"No"* to the sweet menu when you really want one.

As long as you don't eat a gooey sweet every day of your life it is fine to enjoy one when you are out.

On a daily basis you could have:-

Fruit and yoghurt.

You might as well have something that is good for you!

And, no, meringue nests are not good for you – they make you crave sugar even more – trust me!

Are you still hungry?

You must answer this question honestly.

PUDDINGS!

Here at SMART if we need a chocolate fix, we melt Green & Blacks Organic 70% cocoa plain chocolate and coat strawberries or banana pieces with the chocolate and finally dip the chocolate fruit in flaked almonds. Not an E number in sight and they are really quite delicious!

Or:-

We make All-bran tea bread. A very old recipe from Kellogg's using Kellogg's All-bran.

1 cup All-bran
1 cup mixed fruit
¼ cup caster sugar
1 cup milk or tea

Soak all these ingredients overnight. Mix in 1 cup of self-raising flour and place in a greased loaf tin.

Bake for 2 hours at 150c/300f/gas 2.

A slice of this will keep you going for ages!

Shopping List Guide

FRESH FRUIT/VEGETABLES

Seasonal vegetables for soups and evening meals
Salad vegetables – whatever you fancy
Garlic
Onions
Mushrooms
Lemon
Fresh herbs
Fruit – desired choice

DAIRY

Skimmed or semi-skimmed milk
Low-fat bio or Greek yoghurt
Cottage cheese

FROZEN

Peas
Prawns and seafood
Summer fruits

OILS & THINGS

Extra virgin olive oil
Balsamic vinegar
Wholegrain mustard
Schwartz season-all
Spices e.g. curry/chilli
Vegetable bouillon
Worcester sauce
Soy (tamari) sauce

CEREALS ETC

Porridge oats
Cereal from breakfast list
Brown basmati rice
Whole-wheat spaghetti/pasta
Beans & pulses
Soya & linseed bread
Eat Natural cereal bars

TINNED AND PACKAGED

Tinned tomatoes
Tomato puree
Tinned tuna in spring water or brine
Sardines or other oily fish
Coconut milk
St. Dalfour no added sugar jam
Crazy Jacks dried apricots (these are preservative free)
Nairns oat cakes
Honey
70% cocoa dark chocolate
Flaked almonds
Mixed nuts and seeds
Free-range eggs

Conversion Tables

WEIGHT	.
Ounces (oz)	Grams (g)
0.5	15
1	25
1.5	45
2	55
2.5	70
3	85
4	115
5	140
6	170
7	200
8	225
12	340
1lb 8oz	455
1lb 8oz	680
2lb	910

LIQUIDS	.
Fl.oz (pints)	Millilitres (litres) ml
2	60
3	90
4	120
5 (0.25 pint)	140
6	180
7	205
8	230
10 (0.5 pint)	290
12	340
14	400
15	430
20 (1 pint)	570
2 pints	1.11 litres

OVEN TEMPRETURES		
Degrees C	Gas Mark	Fahrenheit
140	1	275
150	2	300
170	3	325
180	4	350
190	5	370
200	6	400
220	7	425
225	8	450

1 tablespoon =	0.5fl.oz/15ml
American pint =	16fl.oz
English pint =	20fl.oz

Kim G Bryan

EXERCISE

Obesity is steadily increasing and this is sadly apparent in the youth of today.

Eating habits are definitely to blame but another reason is definitely a lack of exercise. Today's modern life is full of wonderful gadgets opposed to the lives of our parents and grandparents. My Mother remembers washday being just that, a whole day! They probably expended more energy on this day than many of us do in a week! Cars have replaced bicycles and walking, elevators have replaced stairs (well, stairs are still there but the elevator looks easier!), and play stations and computers have replaced the art of conversation and so on. Basically, the population is turning into couch potatoes!

Little or no exercise leads to less calories being burned and messes up the body's appetite mechanism.

Believe it or not, exercise actually suppresses the appetite hence people who do no exercise whatsoever, have exaggerated appetites!

Crash dieting and very low calorie regimes encourage the body to lose muscle mass.

Muscle burns up more energy than fat, one pound of lean muscle burns 60-70 calories per day opposed to one pound of fat which burns only 10.

Less muscle means more fat and induces a slow metabolism.

THESE DIETS ARE NOT WINNERS!

The metabolic rate is 'like a fire'. Years of yo-yo dieting can extinguish the fire and it can take a very long time to re-light.

THE BENEFITS OF EXERCISE

> ➢ **Exercise has a great effect on metabolism. During a brisk walk or cycle people can raise their resting metabolic rate up to ten times faster and this can be sustained for up to fifteen hours after a session.**

> ➢ **Normalises appetite mechanisms.**

> ➢ **Improves insulin sensitivity.**

> ➢ **Exercise releases chemicals called endorphins that make you 'feel good'.**

Exercise brings about so many benefits that you may wonder why you haven't started sooner.

You do not have to be fanatically fit to benefit from exercising. The important thing to remember is not to become obsessed about it. You can become more active without joining a gym.

> ➢ **Walk up town instead of taking the car.**

> ➢ **Use the stairs instead of elevator lifts.**

> ➢ **Take up an active hobby.**

> ➢ **Start with just fifteen minutes per day or thirty-five minutes three times a week doing exercise you**

enjoy which slightly raises your heart rate. If you have any concerns about starting an exercise regime, consult your doctor.

➢ Combine cardiovascular exercise (walking, running, swimming, aerobics, cycling etc.) with toning/resistance exercise – this helps to build muscle. There are many good DVDs on the market which explain everything in detail and can be carried out in your home.

➢ You will soon find that fifteen minutes per day turns into forty-five and your body will thank you for it.

➢ Try not to overdo it!

➢ If you decide to join a gym, you will be in safe hands. Ask for a training programme to suit you.

➢ Exercise is accumulative. A little each day adds up to an impressive weekly total.

➢ Remember to eat and drink after an exercise session (light meal to replenish energy stores and water to prevent dehydration).

➢ Get out in the fresh air and enjoy a walk.

➢ In my opinion, walking is the best exercise. It's free! And all that fresh air will make you feel so much better.

➢ Recent research with groups of human guinea pigs showed that the participants who walked just thirty minutes daily lost the most weight and also kept the weight off.

Beginning is sometimes the biggest problem!

GET MOTIVATED!

Activities/calorie burning

ACTIVITY	Approximate calories burned in 30 mins*
Aerobics	**211**
Cycling	140
Cross-trainer	180
Dancing	120
Housework	120
Gardening	176
running (9 minute mile)	387
rowing	180
Swimming	211
Tennis	246
Trampette (rebounding)	108
walking (briskly)	140
walking up hill	184

Exercise can easily be incorporated into a normal day.

*This is very approximate as it depends on weight, effort and fitness level of each individual

Kim G Bryan

PSYCHOLOGICAL TROUBLES

There is a saying; *"do you eat to live or live to eat!"*

Food has become a cure for boredom, a release for stress or just a regular habit whilst watching television.

Eating patterns seem to fall in line with the state of your self esteem, as detailed in Chapter One. Life throws many spanners into the works and if food is your answer to this, either by bingeing or starving, it will create problems with weight and also health.

> ➢ **Boredom eating**

We all get bored from time to time and reach for something to relieve this. The trouble is it is so easy to open the cupboard, reach for a packet of biscuits and eat the lot!

Certain situations initiate this urge to eat and it normally has nothing to do with hunger!

The key is to identify these situations e.g. nibbling at night after the evening meal and either occupy yourself or prepare alternative "healthy" nibbles for these times e.g. fruit.

> ➢ **Stress eating**

The solution for stress eating, although it is easier said than done, is to pin point the reason and eradicate it.

If the stress is a result of the weight problem you can begin to make positive changes but you may need help from your Doctor or a counsellor in certain situations.

> ## Habit eating

We are all creatures of habit!

It is very easy to get into a pattern of habit eating e.g. watching television or raiding the fridge when you return home after a working day.

Habits can be automatically built into our daily routines without us being fully aware.

Example: if you visit a newsagent daily to buy your paper. Do you often pick up food as well?

The types of food on sale at these places tend to be the foods that are eaten quickly and then forgotten about!

> ## Cravings

Craving certain foods is another psychological problem. Do you crave through hunger or just the fact that these foods make you feel better?

Chocolate is the number one culprit here. Chocolate is everywhere and is often associated with a certain 'feel good factor!'.If you crave chocolate before your monthly period it is a cry for energy and also magnesium. The thought of never eating chocolate bar again can lead to many emotional troubles including depression and deprivation. If you need chocolate, go ahead and eat it and don't feel guilty about it. The bottom line is you need to take control of your eating. A treat of chocolate now and again will not sabotage your diet but the crazy feelings associated with it will.

> ## Support

Support from family, friends and work colleagues is paramount. People may be negative about your new regime. Do not let any negative comments put you off, they come from people who are just too lazy to change their eating habits or from people who have no idea how to. Focus on your target at all times. If you have a considerable amount of weight to lose, split the weight up into half stones. Each half a stone will make you closer to your target.

> ## Weighing scales obsession

Do not keep hopping on and off the scales! Weight fluctuates throughout the day. Too much emphasis is put on weekly weight loss and this can make people very dejected when weight loss is very small or not at all.

Weigh yourself either once a fortnight or monthly.

A better way of calculating weight loss is to keep an item of clothing aside that is either too tight or just doesn't fit you. Each month, try it on and see how much better it looks and feels.

> ## Choosing the right clothing

Coco Chanel once said;

"Fashion fades and only style remains."

Fashion is changing all the time.

ASK YOURSELF THIS:-

"Do I want to look fashionable or do I want to look good in my clothes?"

Clothes can disguise bulges, make you appear taller and flatter even the fullest of figures.

Many mistakes are made with the clothes we wear.

➢ **Wear clothes that fit you well. Squeezing into clothes that really don't fit will make you look bigger. If you know for sure that one day, you will fit into these clothes again, keep them. If the answer is no, get rid of them. Buying a size ten will not necessarily make you that size!**

➢ **There are many guidelines regarding flattering clothes. Shop with an honest friend or ask the shop assistants.**

Magazines often write articles about clothes and body shapes. Carole Jackson's book Colour me beautiful offers fully explained advice about clothes, colour, make-up etc. If you have no idea, this book is for you.

TROUBLESHOOTING

If you follow all the guidelines in this book, have increased your exercise and your weight/size has not decreased, what do you do?

Check with your GP that you do not have a medical condition which is causing the weight gain.

➢ **Under active thyroid**

There are many symptoms of an under active thyroid (hypothyroidism); feeling cold, depressed, tired, lack of energy, weight gain, dry hair and skin, constipation, menstrual problems and headaches.

From time to time we all get these symptoms in one form or another.

Your GP can arrange a blood test and if an under-active thyroid is detected the correct treatment can be given.

Other problems are:-

- ➢ **Water retention**
- ➢ **Menopause**
- ➢ **Stress and depression**
- ➢ **Medication**
- ➢ **Psychological problems**

Be honest with yourself and don't try and match the symptoms to your weight problem.

If you do have an underlying medical problem your GP will be able to offer support and any treatment needed.

INTOLERANCES AND ALLERGIES

These affect many people and cause much discomfort and in some cases, ongoing illness.

To determine whether you are intolerant to a food you need to check with your GP and the appropriate test can be carried out, or alternatively, visit a professional who specialises in that field.

Allergies to food are far more complex and in certain cases, life threatening.

LACTOSE INTOLERANT

Basically, a person has a shortage of the enzyme lactase and is unable to break down the sugar, lactose into glucose, found in milk and milk products. These shortages can vary dramatically e.g. one person may produce enough lactase to cope with a glass of milk and another may suffer from just one lick of ice-cream.

Common symptoms

> **Nausea**
> **Stomach cramps and bloating**
> **Diarrhoea & severe wind**

These symptoms would normally appear approximately 1-2 hours after eating milk protein or food containing milk proteins.

On the other end of the scale is milk allergy.

This allergy is caused when the immune system reacts against the proteins found in milk. Basically, the immune system views these proteins as harmful and reacts against the protein to destroy it in order to protect the body.

Milk allergy reactions can be seen as itchy red skin and hives, swelling of lips, mouth, tongue and throat, severe bloating and runny diarrhoea, sickness, sneezing, coughing and a shortness of breath. These symptoms will appear within 20 minutes of eating milk protein.

These symptoms are seen in other food allergies. Common food allergies include; seafood, peanuts, eggs and bananas.

CELIAC DISEASE

Celiac disease is also known as gluten intolerance. The disease is, by definition, a condition in which the wall of the intestines becomes damaged as a result of eating gluten. Gluten is found in wheat, rye, barley and oats. There are numerous symptoms for celiac disease ranging from severe abdominal pain to depression.

If you constantly suffer after eating i.e. diarrhoea, nausea, stomach pains etc. consult your GP and he or she will be able to help you diagnose the problem.

Alternatively, you can order an allergy testing kit from Yorktest laboratories.

Yorktest Laboratories Ltd
Murton Way
Osbaldwick
York
YO19 5US

Telephone: 01904 410410
www.allergy.co.uk

All they need us a simple pinprick of blood. Price from £19.99.

Kim G Bryan

KEEPING TRACK OF PROGRESS

Here are a few charts and diaries to help you along the way with your new regime.

It is a good idea to keep a food diary. A diary can highlight problems and help you with food choices when you are not sure what to eat.

Here is an example of a food diary format.

Food Diary

Date:	Date:
Breakfast:	Breakfast:
Lunch:	Lunch:
Evening Meal:	Evening Meal:
Snack:	Snack:
Exercise:	Exercise:
Problems (negative Feelings):	Problems (negative Feelings):
Positive Feelings:	Positive Feelings:

Good Luck and - remember to be honest. You are only kidding yourself if you omit to write something down!

PROGRESS CHARTS

DATE	WEIGHT LOSS	WEIGHT

MEASUREMENTS

This chart will really help you to see the difference. It's not about weight, it's about losing inches, and you'll soon be able to track exactly how your body shape is changing.

Use a tape measure to measure the body parts shown in the table below. The tape measure should be against the skin and not pulled tight.

Date	Date	Date
Bust	Bust	Bust
Waist	Waist	Waist
Hips	Hips	Hips
Buttocks	Buttocks	Buttocks
Left U/Arm	Left U/Arm	Left U/Arm
Right U/Arm	Right U/Arm	Right U/Arm
Left Thigh	Left Thigh	Left Thigh
Right Thigh	Right Thigh	Right Thigh
Left Knee	Left Knee	Left Knee
Right Knee	Right Knee	Right Knee

EXPERT REFERENCES

GI is a proven science.

Various research teams all over the world have tested the concept of GI and how it can help weight control and health.

A SYNOPSIS FROM A STUDY AT OXFORD BROOKES UNIVERSITY.

BREAKFAST 'CURE' FOR CHILDHOOD OBESITY.

Eating the right type of breakfast may be the key to tackling the increasing problem of obesity in children, new research claims.

A study of British youngsters aged 9-12 looked at the effect of different foods on their hunger levels during the day. The children were given meals measured using the Glycaemic Index (GI), which compares the rise in blood glucose levels after eating different foods.

The researchers, from Oxford Brookes University, found that the children who had a low GI breakfast had 'significantly lower lunch intake' compared to those who had a high GI meal.

It is hoped the research could be used to help dieticians prescribe the most effective diet to help combat childhood obesity so that they eat foods that release sugar steadily across the day rather than 'quick fix snacks'.

The low GI breakfast consisted of cereals like bran, muesli, porridge or soya and linseed bread, all with a GI value of less than 55. The high GI breakfast included cornflakes, chocolate flavoured cereal or white bread all with GI values between 75 and 100.

Not only were the high GI group more likely to feel hungry between meals, they also ate more for lunch, the researchers found.

THE PRESS AND JOURNAL, TUESDAY 4TH NOVEMBER 2003.

I asked Thomas Wolever PhD, an expert in the glycaemic index, how he would summarise the benefits of adopting a low GI diet and also how it would benefit health in the long term.

He replied *"Using more low GI foods is a good idea, and may have a wide range of benefits from helping to control body weight to reducing risk for diabetes, heart disease and cancer."*

"A low glycaemic index (low-GI) diet can lead to weight loss, reduced body fat percentages and reduce the risk for diabetes and cardiovascular disease."

A team of researchers from The Harvard Medical School in Boston, USA studied 21 rats and the effects of high GI carbohydrates within their diet opposed to low GI carbohydrates over a period of 18 weeks.

The rats were split into two groups and fed a diet made up of 69% carbohydrate. Both groups of rats were fed in a controlled way that kept their body weight the same throughout the 18 week study.

After 18 weeks the high GI carbohydrate group had 71% more body fat and 8% less lean body mass than the group that were fed low GI carbohydrates.

The high GI carbohydrate group also had significantly greater increases in blood glucose, insulin levels and triglyceride (fat in the blood which greatly increases the risk of heart disease). In fact, the triglyceride levels were nearly three times that of the low GI group.

A further experiment was carried out on 24 mice. The mice were fed either a high or low GI diet. After nine weeks, the high GI group had 93% more body fat that the mice on the low GI diet.

It was also reported that the high GI group required less food to gain the same body weight.

Dr. David Ludwig, MD, PhD, who led the team of researchers, concluded that the study showed how concentrating on eating low GI carbohydrates could have a dramatic effect on major chronic diseases – obesity, diabetes and heart disease.

He also believes that a low glycaemic index diet may be as or more effective than the standard reduced fat diet for weight loss.

REFERENCES & BIBLIOGRAPHY

Processed Food vs. Natural
Glenville, M. (1999) Natural alternatives to dieting London, Kyle Cathie Ltd p46.

The Dangers of Dieting
Holford, P. (1999) The 30 day fat burner diet London, Judy Piatkus (publishers) Ltd p16.

The Glycaemic Index
Jenkins, D. 1981.

The Glycaemic Load
Invented by researchers at Harvard University, Walter Willet.

Kim G Bryan

ABOUT THE AUTHOR

Kim Bryan studied as a weight management consultant at Stonebridge Health College. She is also a qualified beauty therapist and sports massage therapist. Kim owns and runs her own beauty salon in Boston, Lincolnshire. While Kim was studying her diploma she decided to research the glycaemic index. She said, *"It made so much sense to me"*. Kim adopted a low GI diet herself, making small changes and now, it has become a way of life. Once upon a time she did weigh over 13 stone! She has ironed out all the technical bits and re-iterated the diet into an easy, user-friendly guide.

Kim has tried many different diets over the years but found many problems the biggest issue was feeling deprived and hungry.

Kim's SMART GI Diet Plan is easy to implement and you can live with it forever.

DISCLAIMER

The advice offered in The SMART GI Diet Plan is based on current expert opinion and intended for persons who are in good health. It is not a prescriptive or therapeutic diet. It is the responsibility of the reader to seek professional medical advice as appropriate with regard to pre-existing medical conditions.

www.ingramcontent.com/pod-product-compliance
Lightning Source LLC
Chambersburg PA
CBHW070353290526
45790CB00004B/1468